...ctical Management of Depression in Older People

Edited by

Stephen Curran BSc(Hon) MB ChB MRCPsych MMed PhD
Consultant in Old Age Psychiatry, Fieldhead Hospital,
Wakefield; Honorary Senior Lecturer in Old Age Psychiatry,
University of Leeds, Leeds, UK

John P Wattis MB ChB FRCPsych DPMEng
Consultant Psychiatrist, Huddersfield NHS Trust and
Professor of Old Age Psychiatry,
University of Huddersfield, Queensgate, Huddersfield, UK

Sean Lynch MB ChB MRCPsych PhD
Senior Lecturer in Psychiatry, Division of Psychiatry
and Behavioural Sciences in Relation to Medicine,
St James's University Hospital, Leeds, UK

ARNOLD

A m

D0269420

First published in Great Britain in 2001 by
Arnold, a member of the Hodder Headline Group,
338 Euston Road, London NW1 3BH

http://www.arnoldpublishers.com

© 2001 Arnold

British Library Cataloguing in Publication Data
A catalogue record for this book is available from the British Library

ISBN 0 340 76386 8

1 2 3 4 5 6 7 8 9 10

Publisher: Georgina Bentliff
Production Editor: James Rabson
Production Controller: Bryan Eccleshall
Cover Design: Terry Griffiths

Typeset in 10pt Palatino by J&L Composition Ltd, Filey, North Yorkshire
Printed and bound in Great Britain by MPG Books Ltd, Bodmin, Cornwall

What do you think about this book? Or any other Arnold title?
Please send your comments to feedback.arnold@hodder.co.uk

Contents

List of Contributors

Maggie Bell RGN RMN Post Grad Dip Human Ageing
Assistant Director of Organisational Development
Wakefield and Pontefract Community Health NHS Trust, Fieldhead Hospital,
Wakefield, UK

Susan M. Benbow MB ChB MSc FRCPsych Diploma in Family Therapy
Consultant Psychiatrist, Old Age Psychiatry, Central Manchester Healthcare
NHS Trust, Carisbrooke Resource Centre, Manchester, UK

Peter C.W. Bowie MD MMedSc MRCPsych
Senior Lecturer in Old Age Psychiatry, University of Leeds, Division of
Psychiatry, Leeds, UK

Wendy Burn MMed Sc MRCPsych
Consultant Psychiatrist, Psychiatry of Old Age and Associate Medical Director
for Doctors in Training, Newsam Centre, Seacroft Hospital, Leeds, UK

Alan Butler BA (Hons) MA Dip Psychother
Chair of Division of Psychiatry and Behavioural Sciences, School of Medicine,
University of Leeds, UK

Stephen Curran BSc(Hon) MB ChB MRCPsych MMed PhD
Consultant in Old Age Psychiatry, Fieldhead Hospital, Wakefield; Honorary
Senior Lecturer in Old Age Psychiatry, University of Leeds, Leeds, UK

Philip Heywood MB ChB FRCGP DCH DObst RCOG
Professor of Primary Care Development, School of Medicine, University of
Leeds, Leeds, UK

Philip Hughes RMN RGN DPSN BSc(Hons) MBA
Clinical Manager, Mental Health Services for Older People, Wakefield and
Pontefract Community Trust, Ossett Health Centre, Ossett, UK

Sean Lynch MB ChB MRCPsych PhD
Senior Lecturer in Psychiatry, Division of Psychiatry and Behavioural Sciences
in Relation to Medicine, St James's University Hospital, Leeds, UK

Carol Martin MA MSc DipPsych C.Psychol AFBPsS
Lecturer in Clinical Psychology, University of Leeds, Division of Psychiatry
and Behavioural Sciences, Leeds, UK

Gail Mountain Dip COT MPhil PhD
Research and Development Officer, College of Occupational Therapists,
Leeds, UK

Graham P Mulley DM FRCP
Professor of Medicine for the Elderly, St James's University Hospital, Leeds, UK

Martin Neal RMN BSc(Hons) DipN DMS MA
Clinical Nurse Adviser/Research Fellow, Leeds Community Health Trust, Meanwood Park Hospital, Leeds, UK

John P Wattis MB ChB FRCPsych DPMEng
Consultant Psychiatrist, Huddersfield NHS Trust and Professor of Old Age Psychiatry, University of Huddersfield, Queensgate, Huddersfield, UK

Simon Wilson MRCPsych MMedSc BM BS
Consultant in Old Age Psychiatry, High Royds Hospital, Leeds, UK

Getting the measure of depression in old age

John P. Wattis

Introduction

Depression is a disabling and sometimes fatal illness in old people. Those who suffer from it report that severe depression changes life completely. It affects behaviour, relationships, emotions, motivation, thinking, sleep and other somatic functions. The person who could mix well socially suddenly becomes isolated and reclusive. Everything is too much trouble. Personal appearance is neglected and the capacity for enjoyment is attenuated or disappears. Appetite is down, food is not enjoyed and weight is lost. Often sleep is disrupted and waking early in the morning may be compounded by diurnal variation of mood. Severe depression reduces motivation and slows mind and body. Often it distorts thinking and even memories, resulting in pre-occupation with negative themes such as poor physical health, guilt, self-reproach and unworthiness. Agitation sometimes complicates depression and may paralyse the patient's capacity to make decisions or manifest itself in constant seeking for comfort and reassurance. Weepiness is more common in women than men but is often reported indirectly by friends, relatives and carers since the patient may feel she has to conceal her true feelings from strangers. Depression may be fatal indirectly through its interaction with physical illness or directly as a cause of suicide.

Suicide rates for men are higher than for women in a variety of cultural settings and in all age groups. Male suicide rates show two peaks: one in young adulthood and one in old age (Snowdon 1997). The rate in young men has been rising markedly in some cultures but in most settings the peak for old men remains higher. Young male rates in a recent study in the UK from an inner city environment have shown a young male suicide rate higher than that for older men (Neeleman et al. 1997).

Apart from its impact on individuals and their families, depression also has a major impact on the health and social services. Depression is associated with increased mortality (Murphy et al. 1988, Pulska et al. 1999) and depression is more common amongst elderly acute medical inpatients (Burn et al. 1993), among disabled isolated elders (Prince et al. 1997b) and in residential settings (Mann et al. 1984). It contributes to morbidity, mortality and increased usage of non-psychiatric medical services (Beekman et al. 1997). Depression may become more prevalent with increasing age, probably because of an association with disabling and handicapping physical conditions (Roberts et al. 1997). Perhaps partly because of this, it is much more likely to lead to the need for inpatient care. Factors which may contribute to the relatively high hospitalization rate for depression in old age may be summarized as follows:

- factors related to the severity of the depression – including problems in early diagnosis and treatment;
- suicide risk;
- living alone – 31% men and 58% women over 75 years live alone;
- loneliness;
- associated physical illness and disability; and
- association with cognitive impairment in some.

People with depression tend to be heavy consumers not only of inpatient psychiatric facilities but also of inpatient general hospital beds and, in the community of mental health, primary care and social services. No detailed analysis has been made of the economic impact of depression in old age. One comparative study found that dementia was the most expensive disorder per sufferer in terms of services used but that those with depression were also high users of health services. Despite presenting to health services (often 'in disguise'!) most depression remains untreated. The most significant predictors of service cost in a multivariate analysis were living alone, being physically ill, depression, dementia and increasing age (Livingston et al. 1997). Depression stands out as a treatable but relatively untreated condition leading to high consumption of health resources.

In this chapter the prevalence of depression in old age and its associations with other diagnoses, disabilities, handicaps and social factors is considered.

Depressive disorder is essentially treatable but under-diagnosed and under-treated in many different settings (Baldwin 1988, Koenig *et al.* 1988, Murphy *et al.* 1988, Green *et al.* 1994, Snowdon *et al.* 1996) and its higher prevalence in particular groups makes people in those groups ideal candidates for early detection and intervention. We will also therefore briefly consider instruments used for screening, diagnosing and measuring outcome in depression.

Classification and definitions

The major international system for classifying diseases (ICD-10 – World Health Organization 1992) groups all mood disorders together under seven main categories as follows:

- F30 – manic episode;
- F31 – bipolar affective disorder (includes recurrent mania);
- F32 – depressive episode;
- F33 – recurrent depressive disorder;
- F34 – persistent mood disorder;
- F38 – other mood disorder; and
- F39 – unspecified mood disorder.

Each category is subdivided according to severity (mild, moderate or severe) and the presence or absence of psychotic symptoms. There are also coding provisions to record the presence or absence of 'somatic' symptoms (anhedonia, mood worse in the morning and early morning waking). This generates up to 30 different categories for depression, though in practice some are more common than others.

Unfortunately, the need for consistency in diagnosis can generate very complicated rules. For example a diagnosis of depressive episode rests on the following:

(a) The syndrome must be present for at least 2 *weeks*, there must be no history of mania and the depression must not be attributable to organic disease or psychoactive substances (the difficulty of this will become evident when we examine associations with physical illness in more detail).

(b) At least *two* of the following three symptoms must be present:
   (1) Depressed mood to a degree that is definitely abnormal for the individual, present for most of the day and for almost every day, and largely uninfluenced by circumstances.
   (2) Loss of interest or pleasure in activities that are normally pleasurable
   (3) Decreased energy or increased fatiguability

(c) At least *four* of the following symptoms:
   (1) Loss of confidence or self-esteem.
   (2) Unreasonable self-reproach or excessive and inappropriate guilt.
   (3) Recurrent thoughts of death or suicide; suicidal behaviour.

(4) Complaints or evidence of diminished ability to think or concentrate, such as indecisiveness or vacillation.
(5) Change in psychomotor activity with agitation or retardation (either subjective or objective).
(6) Sleep disturbance.
(7) Change in appetite.

To be classified as moderate, at least *six* of the symptoms under section (c) must be present and to meet the criteria for severe depression all three from section (b) and at least *five* from section (c) (at least *eight symptoms from (b) and (c) in total*). *Depressive episodes* (F32), whether or not occurring in the context of *recurrent depressive disorder* (F33), are perhaps our main concern in this volume. However, *dysthymia* (F34.1) is also important. It describes people whose outlook is persistently depressed but whose depression is not sufficiently severe or acute in onset to be described as a depressive episode. Anxiety symptoms are often prominent. The relationship between dysthymia and depressive disorder is not exclusive. Dysthymia may follow or complicate a depressive episode and it is not always clear that they represent different conditions either in terms of causation or treatment.

Epidemiologists and others who research into the relationships between depression and other conditions in old age often must resort to less complicated definitions. The main diagnostic classifications (and the rating scales developed from them) have largely been developed in relation to younger adult patients and may not always be applicable to older adults (Weiss *et al.* 1986). In addition epidemiologists have to employ case-finding instruments which may be *mapped* on to diagnostic systems but may employ variable definitions of 'caseness'. *Pervasive depression* has been used as a term to define a level of caseness that defines depression of a type and severity likely to warrant medical or psychological intervention. Depression in epidemiological studies is diagnosed using instruments such as the Geriatric Mental State (**GMS**) (Copeland *et al.* 1976) examination or the Comprehensive Assessment and Replacement Evaluation (**Short-CARE**) (Gurland *et al.* 1984) schedule. Sometimes self-assessment measures such as the Geriatric Depression Scale (**GDS**) (Herrmann *et al.* 1996), the Brief Assessment Schedule for Depression in the Elderly-Cards (**BASDEC**) (Adshead *et al.* 1992) or the Hospital Anxiety and Depression (**HAD**) (Zigmond and Snaith 1983, Kenn *et al.* 1987, Wattis *et al.* 1994 a, b) scale are used. The correspondence between the categories produced by these latter scales and the more rigorous categories of the **ICD-10** (World Health Organization 1992) and the American Diagnostic and Statistical Manual (**DSM-IV**) (American Psychiatric Association 1994), is at times sketchy but even the simplest self-assessment scales like the HAD measure something that can properly be described as depression and that responds to treatment.

Prevalence of depression in older people

Here we need to distinguish carefully between overall prevalence and the prevalence of depression in subgroups who for one reason or another are at higher risk of developing or continuing to suffer from depressed mood. For example, a large-scale epidemiological study using the GMS (Saunders *et al*. 1991) has shown that having *ever* been a heavy drinker (for a period of at least 5 years) increases the relative risk of depression in old age fourfold. These associations are often complicated and difficult to tease out. Overall, *pervasive depression* probably affects around 12 or 13% at any one time (past month 'point' prevalence) (Gurland 1976), but only about 2–3% older people have a depression that would meet the categoric criteria for *depressive episode*. There has long been conflict of opinion about whether depression is more or less common with increasing age. A recent study showed that prevalence of depression increased over the age of 80 years but that this was mostly associated with chronic health problems and functional impairment rather than a direct effect of ageing (Roberts *et al*. 1997) We will now examine the prevalence of depression in different settings, in different ethnic groups, the effect of depression upon mortality, and in association with different illnesses, social factors, disability and handicap.

Depression in different settings

In residential homes (Mann *et al*. 1984) and hospitals (Burn *et al*. 1993) depression is two or three times more common than in the community. An Italian study shows a very high prevalence of 20% 'major' depression, 4% dysthymic disorders and 13% 'atypical' depression in a geriatric day hospital where there was no distinct old age psychiatry service (Turrina *et al*. 1992). A UK study, using the GMS, of people in receipt of Home Care services found the prevalence of depression to be 26%, half of it severe and often not recognized (Banerjee 1993). A follow-up study of older medical inpatients showed that, when physical illness was controlled for, those who were depressed before discharge saw physicians more frequently, were more often hospitalized and more often needed nursing home care than controls without depression (Koenig and Kuchibhatla 1999).

Depression, culture and ethnicity

There have been few studies of the symptomatology, prevalence or outcome of depression by race. One relatively large-scale study suggests there is at least little difference in symptomatology between African–Americans and non-African–Americans (Blazer *et al*. 1998). A European study using the same case-finding methods in a number of different countries found a wide variation in prevalence from 9% in Iceland to 24% in Munich. The difference was even marked between two UK cities, London (17%) and Liverpool (10%) (Copeland *et al*. 1999). Explanations for these differences are only speculative at present.

Depression and mortality

Overall, point prevalence of depressed mood (mostly DSM-III dysthymia) did not predict mortality amongst the elderly in the community when other factors such as high age, gender, smoking, disability, somatic illnesses and number of medications taken was controlled for (Pulska *et al.* 1997). However, depression persisting over 5 years was associated with increased mortality (Pulska *et al.* 1999). Also, given the associations between heart disease and cancer and depression discussed later, there remains a question as to how logical it is to control for physical illness which is itself associated with disability and depression. Another, hospital study, reported later (Herrmann *et al.* 1998) does show an association between depressed mood (measured dimensionally using the HAD) and increased mortality.

Depression and physical illness

One carefully controlled large-scale ($n = 1286$) study with a 4–year follow up has recently shown that older people who report depressive symptoms are at higher risk of subsequent physical decline in simple tests of motor function (odds ratio 1.55; 95% CI 1.02–2.34) (Penninx *et al.* 1998b). For medical inpatients ($n = 454$), high depression scores on the HAD were associated with mortality at 22 months (multivariate odds ratio 1.9; 95% CI 1.2–3.1, $p < 0.01$) (Herrmann *et al.* 1998). Another study of outcome for depressed hospitalized patients with physical disability showed that, on average 47 weeks after discharge, generally depression and disability varied together (Koenig and George 1998), furnishing further evidence of the strong links between depression and disability in old people that will be explored further later. An interesting ethnic difference emerged in this study in that black people tended to have a better outcome for mood regardless of whether or not physical disability improved.

In a Finnish community study, coronary heart disease, physical disability, and widowhood or divorce were associated with self-reported depression in men. In women the association was between history of clinical depression, physical disability and the use of angiotensin-converting enzyme inhibitors and current depression (Ahto *et al.* 1997). A prospective hospital-based study in the USA of people having elective cardiac catheterization for coronary artery disease showed that at the time of catheterization self-reported physical function differed by the number of arteries stenosed, and observer-rated baseline anxiety and depression quartiles. Deterioration in physical function at 1 year was associated with baseline anxiety or depression but not with baseline artery status. Surgical or medical treatment seemed to neutralize the effect of coronary stenosis on physical function at 1 year but not the negative effect of baseline anxiety or depression (Sullivan *et al.* 1997).

Another large-scale study ($n = 4825$) has shown that, after controlling for other known risk factors, depressed mood persisting over 6 years increased the hazard ratio for developing cancer to 1.88 (95% CI 1.13–3.14). This risk was consistent across most kinds of cancer and was not confined to cigarette smokers (Penninx *et al.* 1998a).

A thorough evaluation of 277 patients from 3 to 4 months after an ischaemic stroke (Pohjasvaara *et al.* 1998) found DSM-III-R major depression in 26% and minor depression in a further 14%. Major depression with no explanatory factor apart from stroke was present in 18%. Analysis showed that dependency in daily life was associated with an increased risk of depression (odds ratio [OR] 1.8; 95% CI 1.1–3.1) with an even greater association with major depression (OR 2.9 95% CI 1.6–5.5). Previous episodes of depression were also associated with a markedly increased risk of post-stroke depression. Another survey of stroke and hip fracture survivors living in private households found high levels (41%) of HAD depression or anxiety and of severe or very severe disability (57%). Not surprisingly there was a strong association between severe disability and anxiety ($p < 0.0005$ OR not given) and severe disability and depression ($p < 0.0001$). These authors also looked at the impact of social contact and found that there was a strong association between social contact and lower prevalence of anxiety ($p < 0.01$) or depression ($p < 0.0001$) (Bond *et al.* 1998). Caregivers also may become anxious or depressed following a stroke in the person they look after. Survivors of stroke and their relatives were asked at 6 months to complete the General Health Questionnaire (GHQ – a measure of emotional distress) and the HAD. Over half the carers were in the abnormal range on the GHQ. Caregivers were more likely to be depressed if the patients were severely dependent or emotionally distressed themselves ($p < 0.01$, OR not quoted) (Dennis *et al.* 1998).

A community survey of over 400 elderly people without dementia also found a general association between gait slowing, heart disease and chronic lung disease and self-reported depressive symptoms and poor life satisfaction. In all conditions except heart disease, the effect appeared to be mediated through disability (Broe *et al.* 1998).

Depression is common, though notoriously difficult to diagnose, in Parkinson's disorder (PD). Symptoms such as cognitive slowing (bradyphrenia) are hard to distinguish from psychomotor retardation. One study found major depression in 16.5% and dysthymia and other forms of depression in 25.7% of patients with PD. Low abilities in activities of daily living correlated with the diagnosis of depressive disorder and with high scores on the Hamilton Depression Rating Scale (an observer rating scale commonly used in trials of antidepressants) (Liu *et al.* 1997).

Depression and dementia

A review of depression in dementia estimated 17–30% of patients have depressive symptoms. Depression-related behavioural problems in patients with Alzheimer's dementia are distressing to caregivers. This is reflected by a prevalence of over 75% of depressed mood in those caring for patients with both dementia and depression (Teri 1997). A study of over 1000 older people in a district of Stockholm, Sweden found a surprisingly high prevalence of dementia (28% by DSM-III-R criteria). More importantly for present purposes it found that the prevalence of major depression at around 12% was around three times higher than in the non-demented. Increased disability was associated with major depression in both demented and non-demented subjects (Forsell and Winblad 1998). A French incidence study in which 397 older people with subclinical cognitive impairment were followed up over 3 years found 11% developing dementia without depression and 5% dementia with depression. Those with dementia plus depression showed significantly greater decrements at 3 years in dressing, washing, use of the telephone and continence (Ritchie et al. 1998).

Depression, impairment, disability, handicap and social factors

Conditions such as depression produce impairments of function that result in a loss of ability (disability). The social response (or lack of response) to this can produce handicap. Depression is very common in selected groups of old people with a variety of disabling illnesses (and in those caring for them). Depression is often associated with increased disability and the direction of causality may be both ways. There are also hints in the studies cited above of a protective effect against depression through social contacts. This takes us back to the now classic study by Murphy on the social origins of depression in old age (Murphy 1982). She found an association between severe life events, major social difficulties, poor physical health and the onset of depression. Working class subjects had a higher incidence of depression and this was associated with both poorer health and greater social difficulties. Lack of a confiding relationship (associated with life-long personality traits) increased vulnerability to depression. A more recent large-scale study failed to support some of these findings but it clearly demonstrated a link between declining health, increasing disability and the onset of depression (Kennedy et al. 1990). Further clarification of the relationship between impairment, disability, handicap, depression and social factors is provided by the 'Gospel Oak' series of studies in London. The prevalence of short-CARE 'pervasive' depression in this relatively deprived area was 17%. Impairment, disability and particularly handicap were strongly associated with depression. The adjusted odds ratio for depression in the most handicapped quartile compared with the least was 24.2 (95% CI 8.8–66.6). Adjusting for handicap abolished or weakened most of the associations between depression and social support, income, older age, female gender and living alone (Prince et al. 1997b). When the overarching effect of handicap was put aside there was a moderate association between depression and the number of life events experienced over the previous year. Personal illness, bereavement and theft were reported as the most salient events. There was a stronger relationship between the number of social support deficits and depression. Social support deficits also related to age, handicap, loneliness and the use of home care services. Loneliness was itself associated with depression (OR 12.4 (7.6–20)) (Prince *et al.* 1997a). A follow-up study a year later found that the 1 year onset rate for pervasive depression was 12% and the maintenance rate for those initially depressed was 63%. There was a high mortality rate among depressed people. Disablement, especially handicap, was the strongest predictor of onset of depression. Lack of contact with friends was a risk factor for onset of depression. For men marriage was protective; but for women it was a risk factor. Maintenance of existing depression was predicted by low levels of social support and social participation rather than by disablement (Prince *et al.* 1998).

Detecting depression and measuring outcome

In this section we will not be concerned with diagnostic interview schedules such as the GMS (Copeland *et al.* 1976), Short-CARE (Gurland *et al.* 1984) and others which are largely used in epidemiological research. Nor will we consider in depth observer rater scales such as the Montgomery Asberg Scale (Montgomery *et al.* 1978) and similar scales used largely to rate outcomes in drug trials. We will instead consider short scales that can be used, especially in high risk populations, to enhance the diagnosis of depression and the possibility of using such short scales for the systematic evaluation of outcome in routine clinical practice with depressed old people.

'Screening' for depression in older people

Screening is generally more effective in high risk populations. The geriatric depression scale (GDS) is most widely used for this purpose. It has been validated in a variety of settings, cultures and languages (Montorio and Izal 1996) and a number of short forms have been developed (Lesher and Berryhill 1994, Shah *et al.* 1997, Hoyl *et al.* 1999). The Brief Assessment Scale for Depression Card-sort (BASDEC) (Adshead *et al.* 1992, Loke *et al.* 1996) is a simple card-sort test which has been validated in an inpatient geriatric population. It has a potential advantage in that the questions are repeated in different languages on the reverse of the card but it has not been validated across cultures or different languages. The Even Briefer Assessment Scale for Depression (EBAS-DEP) (Allen *et al.* 1994) is a related scale. As even five questions from the GDS appear reasonably sensitive and specific at least in a setting with a high prevalence (46%) of depression (Hoyl *et al.* 1999), it may be that the value of these scales is as much in prompting clinicians always to ask about depression as in their intrinsic psychometric properties.

Measuring outcome for depression in old people

Patients' self-report is the most obvious way to measure outcome. When a variety of different interviewers are involved, a self-rating scale such as the GDS has obvious advantages in ensuring that the same factors are being considered. The Hospital Anxiety and Depression (HAD) scale, which does not work well as a screening instrument in geriatric inpatients (Davies *et al.* 1993), does however correlate well with more sophisticated measures of severity (Kenn *et al.* 1987, Wattis *et al.* 1994 a) and appears to function well as an outcome measure in depressed elderly psychiatric inpatients (Wattis *et al.* 1994 b).

Conclusions

In this chapter personal and social consequences of depression in old age have been examined as well as the classification of depression and the effect of depression upon mortality in different settings. The association of depression with mortality and morbidity leads to the conclusion that the detection and treatment of depression in late life is very worthwhile and simple, brief self-rating scales can assist both in detection and in measuring the outcomes of intervention. Depression is particularly prevalent in certain settings and in association with particular conditions.

It is important to be vigilant and possibly employ screening for depression in:

• acute general hospital wards;
• residential care settings;
• physical illnesses;
• physical disability and handicap;
• in those who care for people with stroke or dementia and depression.

In some cases depression seems to cause illness (e.g. cancer) or to hinder recovery (e.g. coronary artery disease). In other cases it seems to be the handicap associated with long-standing illness that leads to depression. There is some evidence that good social relationships can protect against onset of depression and reduce the likelihood of depressed mood persisting. Another key message is that depression in old age is rarely treated, pharmacologically, psychotherapeutically or socially though there is good evidence that all these interventions can make a difference.

The first 'take home' message from this chapter is be aware. Depression is common, particularly in those with physical illness and handicap and in those caring for people with these problems (who are by definition likely to be in contact with health and social services). There is no reason to suppose that depression in these people will fail to respond to treatment so the second 'take home' message is be active. Simple problem-solving psychotherapy that can be delivered in day hospitals, social support and antidepressants all help – so make them available to those in need.

Key points

- Be *aware* of depression in old age, particularly in high risk groups.
- Be *active* in detection.
- Make treatment *available* to those in need.

References

Adshead, F., Day Cody, D., and Pitt, B. (1992) BASDEC: a novel screening instrument for depression in elderly medical inpatients. *British Medical Journal*, **305**, 397.

Ahto, M., Isoaho, R., Puolijoki, H., Laippala, P. , Romo, M., and Kivela, S. (1997) Coronary heart disease and depression in the elderly: a population based study. *Family Practice*, **14**, 436–445.

Allen, N., Ames, D., Ashby, D., Bennetts, K., Tuckwell, V., and West, C. (1994) A brief sensitive screening instrument for depression in late life. *Age and Ageing*, **23**, 213–218.

American Psychiatric Association (1994) *Diagnostic and Statistical Manual of Mental Disorders: DSM-IV*, 4th edn. American Psychiatric Association, Washington, DC.

Baldwin, B. (1988) Late life depression: undertreated? *British Medical Journal*, **296**, 519.

Banerjee, S. (1993) Prevalence and recognition rates of psychiatric disorder in the elderly clients of a community care service. *International Journal of Geriatric Psychiatry*, **8**, 125–131.

Beekman, A.T., Deeg, D.J., Braam, A.W., Smit, J.H., and Van Tilburg, W. (1997) Consequences of major and minor depression in later life a study of disability, well-being and service utilisation. *Psychological Medicine*, **27**, 1397–1409.

Blazer, D.G., Landerman, L.R., Hays, J.C., Simonsick, E.M., and Saunders, W.B. (1998) Symptoms of depression among community-dwelling elderly African–American and white older adults. *Psychological Medicine*, **28**, 1311–1320.

Bond, J., Gregson, B., Smith, M., Rousseau, N., Lecouturier, J., and Rodgers, H. (1998) Outcomes following acute hospital care for stroke or hip fracture: how useful is an assessment of anxiety or depression for older people? *International Journal of Geriatric Psychiatry*, **13**, 601–610.

Broe, G.A., Jorm, A.F., Creasey, H., Grayson, D., Edelbrock, D., Waite, *et al.* (1998) Impact of chronic systemic and neurological disorders on disability, depression and life satisfaction. *International Journal of Geriatric Psychiatry*, **13**, 667–673.

Burn, W.K., Davies, K.N., McKenzie, F.R., Brothwell, J.A., and Wattis, J.P. (1993) The prevalence of psychiatric illness in acute geriatric admissions. *International Journal of Geriatric Psychiatry*, **8**, 171–174.

Copeland, J.R.M., Kelleher, J.M., Kellet, J.M., Gowlay, A.J., Gowland, B.J., Fleiss, J.L., *et al.* (1976) A semi-structured clinical interview for the assessment and diagnosis of mental state in the elderly: the Geriatric Mental Status schedule. *Psychological Medicine*, **6**, 439–449.

Copeland, J.R.M., Beekman, A.T.F., Dewey, M.E., Hooijer, C., Jordan, A and Lawlor, B.A. *et al* (1999) Depression in Europe: geographical distribution among older people. *British Journal of Psychiatry*, **174**, 312–321.

Davies, K.N., Burn, W.K., McKenzie, F.R., Brothwell, J.A., and Wattis, J.P. (1993) Evaluation of the Hospital Anxiety and Depression scale as a screening instrument in geriatric medical inpatients. *International Journal of Geriatric Psychiatry*, **8**, 165–169.

Dennis, M., O'Rourke, S., Lewis, S., Sharpe, M., and Warlow, C. (1998) A quantitative study of the emotional outcome of people caring for stroke survivors. *Stroke*, **29**, 1867–1872.

Forsell, Y. Winblad, B. (1998) Major depression in a population of demented and non-demented older people: prevalence and correlates. *Journal of the American Geriatrics Society*, **46**, 27–30.

Green, B.H., Copeland, J.R.M., Dewey, M.E., Sharma, V., and Davidson, I.A. (1994) Factors associated with recovery and recurrence of depression in older people: a prospective study. *International Journal of Geriatric Psychiatry*, **9**, 789–795.

Gurland, B.J. (1976) The comparative frequency of depression in various age groups. *Journal of Gerontology*, **31**, 283–292.

Gurland, B., Golden, R.R., Teresi, J.A., and Challop, J. (1984) The SHORT-CARE: an efficient instrument for the assessment of depression, dementia and disability. *Journal of Gerontology*, **39**, 166–169.

Herrmann, N., Mittmann, N., Silver, I.L., Shulman, K.I., Busto, U.A., Shear, N.H., *et al.* (1996) A validation study of the Geriatric Depression Scale short form. *International Journal of Geriatric Psychiatry*, **11**, 457–460.

Herrmann, C., Brand-Driehorst, S., Kaminsky, B., Leibing, E., Staats, H., and Ruger, U. (1998) Diagnostic groups and depressed mood as predictors of 22–month mortality in medical inpatients. *Psychosomatic Medicine*, **60**, 570–577.

Hoyl, M.T., Alessi, C.A., Harker, J.O., Josephson, K.R., Pietruszka, F.M., Koelfgen, M. (1999) Development and testing of a five-item version of the Geriatric Depression Scale. *Journal of the American Geriatrics Society*, **47**, 873–878.

Kenn, C., Wood, H., Kucyj, M., Wattis, J.P. , and Cunane, J. (1987) Validation of the Hospital Anxiety and Depression Rating Scale (HADS) in an elderly psychiatric population. *International Journal of Geriatric Psychiatry*, **2**, 189–193.

Kennedy, G.J., Kelman, H.R., and Thomas, C. (1990) The emergence of depressive symptoms in late life: the importance of declining health and increasing disability. *Journal of Community Health*, **15**, 93–104.

Koenig, H.G., Meador, K.G., Cohen, H.J., and Blazer, D.G. (1988) Detection and treatment of major depression in older medically ill hospitalised patients. *International Journal of Psychiatry and Medicine*, **18**, 17–31.

Koenig, H.G. and George, L.K. (1998) Depression and physical disability outcomes in depressed medically ill hospitalized older adults. *American Journal of Geriatric Psychiatry*, **6**, 230–247.

Koenig, H.G. and Kuchibhatla, M. (1999) Use of health services by medically ill depressed elderly patients after hospital discharge. *American Journal of Geriatric Psychiatry*, **7**, 48–56.

Lesher, E.L. and Berryhill, J.S. (1994) Validation of the Geriatric Depression Scale-Short Form amongst inpatients. *Journal of Clinical Psychology*, **50**, 256–260.

Liu, C.Y., Wang, S.J., Fuh, J.L., Lin, C.H., Yang, Y.Y., and Liu, H.C. (1997) The correlation of depression with functional activity in Parkinson's disease. *Journal of Neurology*, **244**, 493–498.

Livingston, G., Manela, M., and Katona, C. (1997) Cost of community care for older people. *British Journal of Psychiatry*, **171**, 56–59.

Loke, B., Nicklason, F., and Burvill, P. (1996) Screening for depression: clinical validation of geriatricians' diagnosis, the Brief Assessment Schedule Depression Cards and the 5–item version of the Symptom Check List among non-demented geriatric inpatients. *International Journal of Geriatric Psychiatry*, **11**, 461–465.

Mann, A., Graham, N., and Ashby, D. (1984) Psychiatric illness in residential homes for the elderly: a survey in one London borough. *Age and Ageing*, **13**, 257–265.

Montgomery, S., Asberg, M., Jornestedt, L., Thoren, P. , Traskman, L., McAuley, R. (1978) Reliability of the CPRS between the disciplines of psychiatry, general practice, nursing and psychology in depressed patients. *Acta Psychiatrica Scandinavica* **271**, 29–32.

Montorio, I. and Izal, M. (1996) The Geriatric Depression Scale: a review of its development and utility. *International Psychogeriatrics*, **8**, 103–112.

Murphy, E. (1982) The social origins of depression in old age. *British Journal of Psychiatry*, **141**, 135–142.

Murphy, E., Smith, R., Lindesay, J., and Slattery, J. (1988) Increased mortality rates in late life depression. *British Journal of Psychiatry*, **152**, 347–353.

Neeleman, J., Mak, V., and Wessely, S. (1997) Suicide by age, ethnic group, coroners' verdicts and country of origin. A three year survey in inner London. *British Journal of Psychiatry*, **171**, 463–467.

Penninx, B.W., Guralnick, J.M., Pahor, M., Ferrucci, L., Cerhan, J.R., Wallace, R.B. (1998a) Chronically depressed mood and cancer risk in older persons. *Journal of the National Cancer Institute*, **90**, 1888–1893.

Penninx, B.W., Guralnik, J.M., Ferrucci, L., Simonsick, E.M., Deeg, D.J., and Wallace, R.B. (1998b) Depressive symptoms and physical decline in community-dwelling older persons. *Journal of the American Medical Association*, **279**, 1720–1726.

Pohjasvaara, T., Leppavuori, A., Siira, I., Vataja, R., Kaste, M., and Erkinjuntti, T. (1998) Frequency and clinical determinants of poststroke depression. *Stroke*, **29**, 2311–2317.

Prince, M.J., Harwood, R.H., Blizard, R.A., Thomas, A., and Mann, A.H. (1997a) Social support deficits, loneliness and life events as risk factors for depression in old age. The Gospel Oak project VI. *Psychological Medicine*, **27**, 323–332.

Prince, M.J., Harwood, R.H., Blizard, R.A., Thomas, A., and Mann, A.H. (1997b) Impairment, disability and handicap as risk factors for depression in old age. The Gospel Oak Project V. *Psychological Medicine*, **27**, 311–321.

Prince, M.J., Harwood, R.H., Thomas, A., and Mann, A.H. (1998) A prospective population-based study of the effects of disablement and social milieu on the onset and maintenance of late-life depression. The Gospel Oak Project VII. *Psychological Medicine*, **28**, 337–350.

Pulska, T., Pahkala, K., Laippala, P., and Kivela, S. (1997) Six-year survival of depressed elderly Finns: a community study. *International Journal of Geriatric Psychiatry*, **12**, 942–950.

Pulska, T., Pahkala, K., Laippala, P., and Kivela, S. (1999) Follow up study of long-standing depression as predictor of mortality in elderly people living in the community. *British Medical Journal*, **318**, 432–433.

Ritchie, K., Touchon, J., and Ledesert, B. (1998) Progressive disability in senile dementia is accelerated in the presence of depression. *International Journal of Geriatric Psychiatry*, **13**, 459–461.

Roberts, R.E., Kaplan, G.A., Shema, S.J., and Strawbridge, W.J. (1997) Does growing old increase the risk for depression? *American Journal of Psychiatry*, **154**, 1384–1390.

Saunders, P. A., Copeland, J.R.M., Dewey, M.E., Davidson, I.A., McWilliam, C., Sharma, V., (1991) Heavy drinking as a risk factor for depression and dementia in elderly men: findings from the Liverpool longitudinal community study. *British Journal of Psychiatry*, **159**, 213–216.

Shah, A., Herbert, R., Lewis, S., Mahendran, R., Platt, J., and Bhattacharyya, B. (1997) Screening for depression among acutely ill geriatric inpatients with a short Geriatric Depression Scale. *Age and Ageing*, **26**, 217–221.

Snowdon, J. (1997) Suicide rates and methods in different age groups: Australian data and perceptions. *International Journal of Geriatric Psychiatry*, **12**, 253–258.

Snowdon, J., Burgess, E., Vaughan, R., and Miller, R. (1996) Use of antidepressants, and the prevalence of depression and cognitive impairment in Sydney nursing homes. *International Journal of Geriatric Psychiatry*, **11**, 599–606.

Sullivan, M.D., LaCroix, A.Z., Baum, C., Grothaus, L.C., and Katon, W.J. (1997) Functional status in coronary artery disease; a one year prospective follow up of the role of anxiety and depression. *American Journal of Medicine*, **103**, 348–356.

Teri, L. (1997) Behavior and caregiver burden: behavioral problems in patients with Alzheimer disease and its association with caregiver distress. *Alzheimer Disease and Associated Disorders*, 11 (suppl. 4), S35–S38.

Turrina, C., Siciliani, O., Dewey, M.E., Fazzari, G.C., and Copeland, J.R.M. (1992) Psychiatric disorders among elderly patients attending a geriatric day hospital: prevalence according to clinical diagnosis (DSMIIIR) and AGECAT. *International Journal of Geriatric Psychiatry*, **7**, 499–504.

Wattis, J., Burn, W.K., McKenzie, F.R., Brothwell, J.A., and Davies, K.N. (1994a) Correlation between Hospital Anxiety Depression (HAD) scale and other measures of anxiety and depression in geriatric patients. *International Journal of Geriatric Psychiatry*, **9**, 61–63.

Wattis, J.P. , Butler, A., Martin, C., and Sumner, T. (1994b) Outcome of admission to an acute psychiatric facility for older people: a pluralistic evaluation. *International Journal of Geriatric Psychiatry*, **9**, 835–840.

Weiss, I.K., Nagel, C.L., and Aronson, M.K. (1986) Applicability of depression scales to the old person. *Journal of the American Geriatrics Society*, **34**, 215–218.

World Health Organisation (1992) *The ICD-10 Classification of Mental and Behavioural Disorders: Clinical Descriptions and Diagnostic Guidelines*, World Health Organisation, Geneva.

Zigmond, A. and Snaith, P. (1983) The hospital anxiety and depression scale (HAD). *Acta Psychiatrica Scandinavica*, **67**, 361–370.

Detection, assessment and diagnosis of depression in older people

Wendy Burn and John P. Wattis

Introduction

The diagnosis of depression in all age groups poses special problems. One multi-national study in primary care found that the majority of attenders with depression complained primarily of physical symptoms (41%), pain (37%) or fatigue and sleep problems (12%) (Wittchen *et al.* 1999). There are wide variations in the point at which a clinician will make a diagnosis of depressive illness. It is relatively simple to recognize depression in the retarded or deluded patient who neither eats nor sleeps. At the other end of the spectrum is a person who is cheerful, energetic, with a good appetite and no difficulty sleeping who is clearly not depressed. If mood is seen as a continuum then at some position between these two examples is a point where a person is seen as having clinical depression. This point is relatively arbitrary and varies between clinicians.

The diagnosis of depression in the elderly provides an even greater challenge than in younger patients. The challenge is, perhaps, greatest of all in older men where there may not only be difficulties on the patient's side in expressing feelings but also on the clinician's side in attributing symptoms to depression (Stoppe *et al.* 1999a). Elderly people experience losses in many areas that may affect how they see the world. Turvey *et al.* (1999) found the rate of syndromal depression was nine times higher in recently bereaved people than in those who were married and that in some patients depression persisted for at least 2 years following bereavement. There is also evidence of possible gender differences in response to bereavement (Chen *et al.* 1999) A high prevalence of physical problems due to other causes and a tendency for patients themselves to fail to recognize psychological problems adds to the difficulty.

As yet there are no physical investigations to confirm or deny the presence of depressive illness. Magnetic resonance imaging (MRI) can already delineate a subtype of late onset depression with relatively poor prognosis (O'Brien *et al.* 1998) and there are hints that localized hypo-perfusion seen on MRI scan may characterize some forms of depression associated with cardiovascular disease (Doraiswamy *et al.* 1999). However, for all practical purposes this is one of the last areas of clinical practice where the skills of history taking and examination alone provide the diagnosis.

The point prevalence of major depression in elderly primary care attenders may be as high as 9%, or more (Schulberg *et al.* 1998) so identification is a priority, especially since the prognosis of untreated depression in old age is poor (Sharma *et al.* 1998, Cole *et al.* 1999).

History taking

As with all diagnosis of psychiatric illness the history taking from an elderly person who you suspect may be depressed is of paramount importance. Wherever possible the patient should be interviewed in their *own home*. It is physically easier for the person concerned and less anxiety-provoking than a hospital setting. The environment provides many clues, both obvious and subtle, to the interviewer that will help in the understanding of both the illness's cause and its effect on function.

If possible the history should be taken with only the patient and interviewer present. Where the presence of another person is unavoidable this party should be as unobtrusive as possible. Many elderly people are treated as children by their relatives and carers and the interviewer may need to explain politely that it is best for the initial part of the assessment to be *conducted in private* with an opportunity for relatives to join in later. It is particularly difficult to explore suicidal feelings if there is an 'audience'. One of the authors once tried to explore suicidal feelings in the presence of a medical student, a daughter and two home care assistants and found it almost impossible.

The history begins with an account of the *'presenting complaint'*, or what has brought the person to your attention. Elderly patients are less psychologically minded than younger ones and may not easily describe themselves as depressed. Problems are often seen as physical rather than mental and careful questioning may be needed to elucidate the problem.

The interview should then move on to questions that specifically address the symptoms of *depression*. These should include descriptions of:

- mood;
- interests;
- concentration;
- hopes for the future; and
- ability to enjoy life.

It is common for elderly people with depression to describe their mood as normal while admitting to a loss of interest in their usual pastimes and an inability to concentrate on books, magazines and the television. There may also be social withdrawal and isolation from others. Questions about hope for the future are useful even in the very elderly. An elderly person who is not depressed may show a detachment from the future while one who suffers a depressive illness faces it with fear and anxiety.

While exploring mood the interviewer should look for the presence of *anhedonia*, one of the core symptoms of depression (Snaith 1993). In anhedonia there is a complete loss of the pleasure response, with an inability to enjoy anything. This may be present even in a person who does not see themselves as depressed and may be justified by 'nothing nice ever happens to me'. The presence of this symptom makes a diagnosis of depressive illness virtually certain. The depression part of the Hospital Anxiety and Depression scale (Zigmond and Snaith 1983) is largely constructed around the concept of anhedonia.

Mood may fluctuate with time. Typically mood in depressive illness is low in the morning and improves as the day goes on. In extreme cases the patient may be found lying in bed in the morning, withdrawn and not wishing to eat, while in the evening they appear completely well. Clinicians performing assessments late in the day should be aware of this possibility. It also needs to be borne in mind when assessing patients over a period of time since if assessments are performed at varying times of the day this may not give a true picture of progress.

Other areas to explore in addition to mood are:

- self-esteem;
- self-confidence;
- guilt; and
- irritability.

Irritability is an important symptom of depression that is often overlooked. It is characterized by a lack of ability to control temper and is very stressful for the individual's relatives and carers.

Religious belief and observance has an impact not only on *suicidal behaviour* but also on prognosis for depression (Koenig *et al.* 1998). For these reasons *belief* and *observance* should be explored as part of the psychiatric history.

Depression also has an effect on *sleep*. Sleep disturbance takes a variety of forms with the most characteristic being initial insomnia and early morning wakening. In initial insomnia the patient lies awake for hours after the time that they would usually go to sleep. In early morning wakening the person wakes in the early hours of the morning (often around 4 a.m.) and is unable to sleep again. The presence of early morning wakening is strongly suggestive of depression, but any change in sleep pattern can be due to a depressive illness. Again this may be hard to assess if the patient claims physical reasons, e.g. needing to go to the toilet, for interrupted sleep. The key point about depressive early morning wakening is the failure to go to sleep again. Rarely, the depressed patient may sleep *more* than usual.

Change in *appetite* is another important area to explore. The usual pattern in depression is loss of appetite with associated loss of *weight*, but in some cases over-eating with weight gain may be present.

Once the symptoms of depression have been explored it is usual to move on to personal, or *life history*. This should include biographical details including major events that may have influenced the individual's psyche.

Information should also be collected about:

- past medical history;
- previous psychiatric problems;
- medication;
- family history of psychiatric illness;
- previous personality; and
- social circumstances.

Never forget to ask about *alcohol* consumption as this is a common aetiological factor in depression. The main points that should be covered when taking a psychiatric history are summarized in Table 2.1.

Table 2.1. Taking a psychiatric history.

Reason for referral
History of presenting illness
(Symptoms, length of time they have been present, severity, effect on functioning)
Family history
(Occupation of parents, dates and causes of their deaths, details of siblings, physical and psychiatric illness in family members)
Personal history
(Place of birth, childhood, occupation, marriage, children)
Medical history
(Any medical illness)
Medication
Past psychiatric history
(Dates of illnesses, diagnoses, treatment)
Premorbid personality
Social history
(Living circumstances, help in the home, use of alcohol, hobbies and pastimes)

Mental state examination

The mental state examination is as important an aid to diagnosis as the history. It begins with observations on the patients *appearance* and *behaviour*. Clues to the presence of depression may be obvious neglect with poor hygiene or more subtle changes such as no make-up or jewellery in someone who normally wears these. Depressed people tend to chose dark or drab clothing and avoid colours such as red or orange. Behaviour may reflect agitation, with the patient pacing up and down the room, or there may be psychomotor retardation when movement and *speech* are abnormally slowed. In severe depression the patient may lie in a stupor, with eyes closed and no response to questions.

The mental state examination should also consider *talk* and *thought*. In depression speech may be slow, non-spontaneous and sparse. Thought content will be pessimistic or empty, sometimes preoccupied with worries about health, family or money.

Mood must be assessed both from the patient's and the clinician's point of view. Sometimes these are referred to in medical short hand as '*subjective*' and '*objective*'. Mention has already been made of some elderly people's inability to recognize their own low mood. The interviewer should use their own emotional response as a measure of the individual's mood. Depression is 'infectious', even on short exposures, and if you reach the end of an interview feeling that the patient's life is hopelessly bleak it is likely that you are sensing a depressed mood.

Questions should be used to elucidate symptoms such as *phobias, obsessions* and *compulsions*. These symptoms may appear or worsen in depression and are often hidden by the individual who experiences them.

Psychotic symptoms are found in some cases of severe depression. Auditory hallucinations are likely to be mood congruent and are typically of defamatory or accusatory voices. Delusions are often paranoid or involve ideas of guilt, sin or poverty. There may, for example, be a belief that the individual has been unfaithful to their marital partner when in fact this is untrue. In Cotard's syndrome nihilistic and hypochondriacal delusions are extreme with ideas that internal organs are rotting or absent or that the patient is already dead. Delusional happenings in depression are usually thought to be deserved, in keeping with feelings of guilt and low self-esteem.

An essential part of the mental state examination is exploration of *suicidal ideas*. Despite its importance (Waern *et al.* 1999) this is an area that doctors are reluctant to approach and where improved training is needed (Stoppe *et al.* 1999b). This is a sensitive subject but is best approached openly and frankly. Patients who are horrified and offended by questions of this nature may be harbouring suicidal ideas they may even be concealing from themselves. An open question such as: 'Have things become so bad that you have considered harming yourself?' or, even less threatening, 'Have you ever felt that life is not worth living?' should be used. Those with suicidal ideas must be asked about plans, what methods they have considered and what has stopped them from acting. No psychiatric assessment by any professional can be considered complete until this question has been addressed.

The *cognitive* assessment is naturally an important part of the mental state examination of an older person. It is usual to use a standardized assessment, such as the mini-mental state examination (Folstein *et al.* 1975). Depression may give rise to low scores due to the effect on attention and concentration. Though further investigation is needed in patients with depression and apparent cognitive impairment, the clock-drawing test may, however, be able to discriminate between dementia and depression (Herrmann *et al.* 1998).

Insight can be tested by questions such as 'Do you think you are unwell?' and 'Do you think that any treatment might help you?'. The measurement of insight can help to determine whether the patient is likely to comply with treatment. The mental state examination is summarized in Table 2.2.

Table 2.2. Mental state examination.

Appearance and behaviour
(Grooming, style of dress, movement, sociability)

Talk and thought
(Rate, form and flow of talk. Thought content)

Mood
Clinician's assessment ('Objective')
Patient's assessment ('Subjective')

Thoughts, beliefs and experiences
(Obsessional ideas, phobias, compulsions, delusions, hallucinations)

Suicidal ideas

Cognitive assessment

Insight

Physical illness

The assessment of any patient suspected of being depressed must always include a search for *physical* illness. This involves:

- a brief history of any physical symptoms; and
- a physical examination.

Particular consideration should be given to *medication* as many commonly prescribed drugs can give rise to depressive symptoms. Those most likely to do so include steroids, anti-hypertensives and diuretics. A physical examination is useful, as are simple screening blood tests including full blood count, urea and electrolytes, glucose, liver function tests and thyroid function tests.

Informant history

No psychiatric examination is complete until an *informant* has been interviewed. This may not always be possible (for example, due to availability of informant, time pressure, or refusal from the patient) but is always desirable. Valuable information can be obtained about changes in the patient's behaviour which may suggest depression. These changes often include a loss of interest and reduction in usual pastimes, or social withdrawal. Low mood and accompanying symptoms are sometimes concealed by a person who feels ashamed of them and on occasions it is only by speaking to an informant that the true picture is obtained.

The patient's *permission* must be obtained before discussing them with any third party. Occasionally, in very high risk situations, this ethical rule may be breached.

Atypical presentation of depressive illness

Not all depressive illnesses present in the usual manner, and elderly patients are particularly prone to unusual presentations. *Somatic* complaints and *hypochondriasis* are relatively common (Gurland 1976). Patients may show no obvious signs of low mood, presenting instead with a physical complaint that is difficult to explain. An example of this is summarized in Case History 2.1.

Case History 2.1

Mr A, aged 75, was seen at his home. A previously fit man he had suddenly started to complain that one of his legs was shorter than the other. He could not accept the assurances of several doctors that this was incorrect. He had taken to his bed and was unable to sleep or eat. He attributed this to his worry over his leg and consistently denied any feeling of depression. He appeared mildly agitated in mood but not obviously low. After observation in hospital it was felt that the most likely diagnosis was a depressive illness and he received treatment for this. He made a full recovery and accepted that there was no physical problem with his leg.

Patients such as Mr A will be familiar to all those who work with elderly people with psychiatric problems. Another atypical presentation of depressive illness is cognitive impairment, or *depressive pseudodementia* (Wells 1979). This can be difficult to distinguish from dementia, but must not be missed as with treatment it can be reversed. The patient appears to suffer memory loss and disorientation but with a greater lack of concentration that is found in true dementia. Typically they do not co-operate well with cognitive testing and frequently answer 'don't know' to questions as opposed to providing incorrect answers. If in doubt then a treatment trial is indicated and may produce dramatic effects. However, patients who develop cognitive impairment in the context of depressed mood may be more likely to develop dementia in future and careful reassessment of cognitive function, when the depression is better, is useful. The situation is further complicated by the fact that depressed mood is more common than might be expected by chance in early dementia, especially vascular dementia (Simpson *et al.* 1999). When it occurs, treatment is still indicated and often beneficial.

Another form which depression may take in the elderly is *behavioural disturbance*. A typical example is a person who has frequent *unexplained falls*. These are usually dramatic but rarely result in injury. If the person believes themself to be unobserved they may be seen lowering themselves gently to the ground before claiming that they have fallen. This type of behaviour is an expression of depression in some individuals and this diagnosis should always be considered in such a situation. Such patients should not be dismissed as 'hysterical' and an example of this is summarized in Case History 2.2.

Case History 2.2

Mrs B, a 73-year-old lady was living in a residential home. She was constantly 'falling' and shouting for help. Staff had observed her when she was unaware that they were watching and had seen her deliberately throw herself to the ground. She was referred with the possible diagnosis of personality disorder and was seen by the care staff of the home as behaving in a 'bad' way. On taking a full history she was found to have sleep and appetite disturbance but denied low mood. She was treated with an antidepressant and her behaviour gradually returned to normal. The falling stopped and her appetite and sleep also improved. Unusual behaviour in elderly people should always suggest the possibility of underlying depression.

Assessment of risk

Assessing *suicide risk* is a mandatory part of any psychiatric assessment, especially when depressed mood is suspected. There may be other risks, too. *Self-neglect* is a problem, especially in people living alone. This may involve:

- not eating;
- not drinking;
- neglect of personal hygiene; and
- failure to take necessary medication, including antidepressants.

Very rarely, even in old people, the risk of homicide may arise (Case History 2.3). Various schedules have been developed to help in 'risk assessment' but their chief value probably lies in their ability to prompt the clinician carefully to consider relevant issues rather than in any strong 'predictive' ability.

Case History 2.3

An elderly man whose first language was not English was looked after by his English-speaking wife. When he became depressed he became irritable and suspicious of her and made a half-hearted attack on her with a knife. When his depression was treated his mood improved and the threat to his wife disappeared. However, it was important to keep his treatment and his mood under review as it was judged that the danger might recur if the depression returned.

Assessment as a means of engaging the patient in treatment

The initial assessment may well determine how co-operative the patient will be in any treatment plan suggested by the clinician. An assessment where the clinician shows a genuine *interest* in and *respect* for the patient as well as an understanding of their circumstances is likely to encourage the patient to co-operate. Indeed, when a patient finds the interrogatory nature of a 'standard' medical assessment too threatening, a more empathetic approach, simply reflecting back what the patient says, may be a helpful way of 'unlocking' a stuck interview. The patient (and their carer if appropriate) needs to be engaged in understanding the diagnosis and treatment plan. If medication is to be prescribed, it needs to be explained that beneficial effects are generally delayed and side-effects must be briefly discussed. The clinician must make an assessment of the likelihood of the patient agreeing to and following any agreed treatment plan. If depression is severe and risk is high the patient may have to be persuaded to accept close monitoring at home or intensive day treatment. In the most severe cases, particularly where there are problems with treatment compliance or the patient lives alone, inpatient care may be indicated.

Assessment under the Mental Health Act

The 1983 Mental Health Act is due for revision and only applies to England and Wales. At present it allows people with mental disorder to be admitted to hospital for assessment and treatment in the interests of their own health or safety or in the interests of the safety of others. 'Guardianship' provisions allow the guardian access to the patient in the community, to direct where the patient lives and to require the patient to attend for (broadly defined) treatment. Most of the Mental Health Act provisions require two medical recommendations, one from a doctor approved under section 12 of the Act (usually a consultant or senior trainee in psychiatry) and one from a doctor who has known the patient over a period of time (usually the general practitioner). This is not the place to go into the legal details, but it is important always to consider use of the Mental Health Act or similar legislation in other jurisdictions, as an option where the patient presents a risk to self or others.

Assessment as an ongoing process and teamwork

Although the emphasis throughout this chapter has been on the initial assessment of the patient with depressed mood, people change and assessment has to be carried out repeatedly. Often follow up may be with a community nurse, even when the initial assessment was made by a doctor. In these cases use of scales such as the Hospital Anxiety and Depression (HAD) scale or the Geriatric Depression Scale (GDS) (Yesavage et al. 1983) enable assessments made by one person to be compared with assessments made by another. These are discussed in greater detail in Chapter 1. When people work in teams, it is useful to have a regular review where different team members present patients briefly so that progress can be monitored and help enlisted. If one member of the team is worried about risk of suicide increasing, another member of the team may be able to make an assessment and agree on management (including admission to hospital if necessary) thus sharing the burden of risk assessment. The formal mechanism for management of patients in the community in the UK is described as the 'Care Programme Approach' or 'Care Management'. These involve reviews that go wider than the multi-disciplinary psychiatric team, patient and carers and may also involve general practitioner, social services personnel, and others. Often resource limitations or good practice dictate that a grand meeting of all involved is not the best way to determine care though in some cases, especially where different points of view need to be reconciled, where risk is very high or where there is great complexity, such a meeting may be needed. The kind of multi-disciplinary team review described earlier may often be the most efficient compromise, provided patients, carers and other interested parties are involved in the process, usually through consultation with the 'key worker' in the multi-disciplinary team.

Key points

- Assessment is the core of any therapeutic process.
- Careful, repeated, systematic assessment of mood and risk form the basis for treatment plans.
- Standardized assessments of mood enable comparison between different time points and different clinicians' assessments.
- Assessments need to be shared in care planning whether or not this is done in formal 'care planning meetings'.
- Perhaps most important of all assessment is the process through which clinicians and patients develop a shared view of what is wrong and what can be done to put it right. Assessment is therefore as much about skills in building relationships as about eliciting information for diagnosis and treatment plans.

References

Chen, J.H., Bierhals, A.J., Prigerson, H.G., Kasl, S.V., Mazure, C.M. and Jacobs, S. (1999) Gender differences in the effects of bereavement-related psychological distress in health outcomes. *Psychological Medicine*, **29**, 367–380.

Cole, M.G., Bellavance, F. and Mansour, A. (1999) Prognosis of depression in elderly community and primary care populations: a systematic review and meta-analysis. *American Journal of Psychiatry*, **156**, 1182–1189.

Doraiswamy, P. M., MacFall, J., Krishnan, K.R., O'Connor, C., Wan, X., Benaur, M. *et al.* (1999) Magnetic resonance assessment of cerebral perfusion in depressed cardiac patients: preliminary findings. *American Journal of Psychiatry*, **156**, 1641–1643.

Folstien, N.F., Folstien, S.E. and McHugh, P. R. (1975) Mini-mental state: a practical method for grading the cognitive state of patients for the clinician. *Journal of Psychiatry Research*, **12**, 189–198.

Gurland, B.J. (1976) The comparative frequency of depression in various adult age groups. *Journal of Gerontology*, **31**, 283–292.

Herrmann, N., Kidron, D., Shulman, K.I., Kaplan, E., Binns, M., Leach, L. *et al.* (1998) Clock tests in depression, Alzheimer's disease, and elderly controls. *International Journal of Psychiatry in Medicine*, **28**, 437–447.

Koenig, H.G., George, L.K. and Peterson, B.L. (1998) Religiosity and remission of depression in medically ill older patients. *American Journal of Psychiatry*, **155**, 536–42.

O'Brien J., Ames D., Chiu E., Schweitzer I., Desmond P. and Tress B. (1998) Severe deep white matter lesions and outcome in elderly patients with major depressive disorder: follow up study. *British Medical Journal*, **317**, 982–984.

Schulberg, H.C., Mulsant, B., Schulz, R., Rollman, B.L., Houck, P. R. and Reynolds, C.F., 3rd. (1998) Characteristics and course of major depression in older primary care patients. *International Journal of Psychiatry in Medicine*, **28**, 421–36.

Sharma, V.K., Copeland, J.R., Dewey, M.E., Lowe, D. and Davidson, I. (1998) Outcome of the depressed elderly living in the community in Liverpool: a 5–year follow-up. *Psychological Medicine*, **28**, 1329–1337.

Simpson S., Allen H., Tomenson B. and Burns A. (1999) Neurological correlates of depressive symptoms in Alzheimer's disease and vascular dementia. *Journal of Affective Disorders*, **53**, 129–136.

Snaith, R.P. (1993) Anhedonia: a neglected symptom of psychopathology. *Psychological Medicine*, **23**, 957–966.

Stoppe, G., Sandholzer, H., Huppertz, C., Duwe, H. and Staedt, J. (1999a) Gender differences in the recognition of depression in old age. *Maturitas*, **32**, 205–212.

Stoppe, G., Sandholzer, H., Huppertz, C., Duwe, H. and Staedt, J. (1999b) Family physicians and the risk of suicide in the depressed elderly. *Journal of Affective Disorders*, **54**, 193–198.

Turvey, C.L., Carney, C., Arndt, S., Wallace, R.B. and Herzog, R. (1999) Conjugal loss and syndromal depression in a sample of elders aged 70 years or older. *American Journal of Psychiatry*, **156**, 1596–1601.

Waern, M., Beskow, J., Runeson, B. and Skoog, I. (1999) Suicidal feelings in the last year of life in elderly people who commit suicide [letter]. *Lancet*, **354**, 917–918.

Wells, C.E. (1979) Pseudodementia. *American Journal of Psychiatry*, **136**, 895–900.

Wittchen, H.U., Lieb, R., Wunderlich, U. and Schuster, P. (1999) Comorbidity in primary care: presentation and consequences. *Journal of Clinical Psychiatry*, **60** (Suppl. 7), pp. 29–36.

Yesavage, J.A., Brink, T.L., Rose, T.L., Lum, O., Huang, V., Adey, M. *et al.* (1983)

Development and validation of a geriatric depression screening scale; a preliminary report. *Journal of Psychiatric Research*, **17**, 37–49.

Zigmond, A.S. and Snaith, R.P. (1983) The hospital anxiety and depression scale. *Acta Psychiatrica Scandinavica*, **67**, 361–370.

The prognosis of depression in later life

Peter Bowie

Introduction

The outcome of depression in old age can be considered in a number of ways. First, what is the natural course of the illness? Second, can the course be modified in the short term, is there a response to specific interventions? Third, what is the longer-term outcome of the disorder in terms of resolution of symptoms, death, or other disability such as dementia. These outcomes have been the subject of scientific investigation; other outcomes such as quality of life, use of resources, functional level, dependency and social adaptation have to date been neglected. Lastly, what variables present in an individual patient predict a particular outcome? In addition we need to consider whether or not the prognosis in late life is different to the same disorder occurring at an earlier age.

In the last two decades there have been a large number of studies reporting the outcome of depression in old age. The majority followed a study by Murphy (1983) who painted a gloomy picture. She reported the 1–year outcome of elderly depressives was favourable in only 35% of her community sample. This study had a number of flaws, the most notable being the lack of standardized treatment, leading to considerable debate that the sample had been under-treated. Another flaw, but one not addressed by subsequent studies, was that some patients had a prior history of major depression although not in the previous 5 years. Clearly, patients with a history of recurrent disorder will tend to adversely effect longer-term outcome studies. There have been no reports of studies of the outcome of depression with first onset in old age. Other methodological problems frequently found include retrospective designs and a variation in the definition of old age, with some studies including patients from the age of 55 years.

Fortunately, the outcome studies have been systematically reviewed on a number of occasions. The reviews themselves have improved in quality, and most recently have used criteria described by the Evidence-Based Medicine Working Group.

Long-term natural history

Relatively little is known about the natural history of depressive disorders in the elderly, although a number of longitudinal studies of elderly depressives living in the community have been reported in the last decade. The most recent report of Sharma *et al.* (1998) followed-up for 5 years a community sample of elderly people living in Liverpool. A previous community survey of 1070 elderly had identified 120 cases of depression using the Geriatric Mental State structured interview. These cases together with other psychiatric cases and a random sample of non-cases were followed up. Outcomes were described in terms of ongoing depression, organic brain disease and mortality. Twenty-eight per cent of the sample was lost to follow up and 34% died during the 5–year period. The relative mortality of the cases compared with non-cases was 2.1 (95% CI 1.1–3.9). Of the remaining 46 cases who completed the study one-quarter were classed as cases at all of the assessments – the illness had run a chronic course. In addition, about 30% of the drop-outs had remained chronically depressed up to the time that they were lost to follow up. The implication of this and similar studies is that untreated depressive disorder in elderly people living in the community carries a poor prognosis, with an increased risk of death or a chronic depressive state. The authors also note that less than 10% of this sample received antidepressant treatment for their disorder during the study period.

Short-term outcome (response to treatment)

This aspect of outcome has been the subject of a recent systematic review. McCusker *et al.* (1998) reviewed the effectiveness of treatments for elderly depressed patients in an outpatient or community setting. The reviewers searched two electronic databases and manually searched bibliographies. From 233 articles, 37 studies were selected that fulfilled the inclusion criteria (original research, prospective controlled design, subjects 55 years and older, diagnosis and outcome measure of depression, and an acute phase pharmacological or psychological treatment). Treatment was classified into pharmacological (heterocyclic antidepressants, selective serotonin re-uptake inhibitors (SSRIs) and anti-anxiety agents) and psychological. Psychological treatments were sub-classified into rational (cognitive or behavioural therapies) and emotive (dynamic or supportive therapies). For the drug studies the control group received either a comparison drug or placebo; for psychological treatments the control group was either untreated (e.g. on a waiting list) or receiving non-specific similar attention. Quality criteria for methodology and treatment were described and two raters assessed the 37 included studies against these. Quality ratings improved in relation to year of publication. Studies published before 1985 had the lowest rating and those published after 1990 the highest. Twenty-six of the studies involved pharmacological treatment and 14 psychological treatment. Pharmaceutical companies funded the majority of drug studies whereas psychological treatment studies were more often funded by independent grants.

A meta-analysis of outcome comparisons was carried out. Using the Hamilton Depression Rating Scale to assess outcome both the heterocyclic and SSRI drug versus placebo comparisons produced significant post-treatment differences. Anti-anxiety drugs were not significantly better than placebo. When compared with untreated controls emotive treatments were not significantly better. Rational treatments however performed significantly better than untreated controls but not significantly better than the attention controls. The mean improvements in Hamilton Depression Rating Scale scores are listed in Table 3.1.

In conclusion the reviewers comment that only heterocyclic and SSRI drugs are effective in the short term. However the post-treatment difference in severity of depression is rather modest, approximately six points on the Hamilton Depression Rating Scale. As for psychological treatments the rational therapies appear more effective than emotive therapies. Compared with untreated controls a post-treatment difference similar to that seen with drugs was found. However this difference disappeared when the therapy was compared with attention controls, a finding that suggests that attention alone may be an effective treatment in the short term for depression. The modest outcomes that were found in this review may be in part attributable to the treatment duration of the studies, with one in four studies being 4 weeks or less. The reader may therefore conclude that although the studies included in this review were at least of reasonable quality, under-treatment of the illness may be a significant factor in the modest outcome. The issue of under-treatment of depression in old age has been highlighted before (Baldwin 1991).

Table 3.1. Mean improvements in Hamilton Depressing Rating Scale scores

Antidepressant class/drug	Mean change in rating scale scores
Tricyclics	-5.8
Fluoxetine	-2.4
Trazodone	-7.5
Phenelzine	-0.8
Rational therapies	-7.3

Another meta-analysis on the short-term outcome of depression is also worthy of mention. Mittmann *et al.* (1997) carried out a meta-analysis on the efficacy and tolerability of antidepressant drugs used in late life depression. Studies were selected from an initial search of two databases. Inclusion criteria were slightly different to those used by McCusker *et al.* (1998) in that the lower age limit was 60 years, studies had to be at least 4 weeks duration and be double-blind randomized controlled trials. Two reviewers examined over 150 reports and assessed them against inclusion criteria – there was no quality assessment for the inclusion criteria. Two meta-analyses were carried out; the first examined the efficacy and tolerability of each antidepressant class. The second examined comparative studies between antidepressants. Outcome measures were response to treatment (number of subjects with at least a 50% reduction in Hamilton or Montgomery Asberg Depression Rating Scale scores) and tolerability (number of subjects reporting adverse events or dropping out). Most of the studies failed to meet the inclusion criteria. The results

Table 3.2. Response to treatment, adverse events and drop-out rates with different antidepressant groups.

Antidepressant class	Proportion of responders (number of subjects)	Adverse events reported (number of subjects)	Proportion of drop-outs (number of subjects)
Atypical	33.4%(30)	38%(280)	11%(375)
RIMA	not available	58%(106)	27%(96)
SSRI	58%(606)	59%(501)	19%(1373)
Tricyclic	63%(166)	60%(276)	23%(860)
Placebo	27%(302)	40%(111)	26%(476)

RIMA, reversible inhibitor of monoamine oxidase.

Table 3.3. The meta-analysis of antidepressant comparison studies.

Comparison	Difference in efficacy (significance)	Difference in adverse event (significance)	Difference in drop-out rates (significance)
Atypical vs RIMA	No data	-12% (ns)	No data
Atypical vs SSRI	-37% (p = 0.01)	8% (ns)	8% (ns)
Atypical vs tricyclic	No data	No data	1% (ns)
Atypical vs placebo	No data	12% (ns)	-15% (ns)
RIMA vs SSRI	No data	No data	No data
RIMA vs tricyclic	No data	-9% (ns)	11% (ns)
RIMA vs placebo	No data	0%	15% (ns)
SSRI vs tricyclic	3.3%	-10% (ns)	-4% (ns)
SSRI vs placebo	14% (ns)	No data	3% (ns)
Tricyclic vs placebo	No data	37% (ns)	1% (ns)

RIMA, reversible inhibitor of monoamine oxidase.

for those studies included in the meta-analyses are set out in Tables 3.2 and 3.3.

The reader can make a number of conclusions from the data presented. Firstly, the short-term outcome of depression in old age is improved by antidepressants. The placebo response (50% reduction in depression scores) rate of 27% is similar to other studies and is substantially less than the response rates for tricyclic and SSRI antidepressants. However, in comparative studies there is no statistical evidence that either of these two drug classes are superior to placebo when using this outcome – this may be a reflection of the number of patients involved in the studies suitable for the meta-analysis. Despite the lack of statistical evidence the reader could reasonably assume that the efficacy differences cited in Table 3.2 represent a clinically important difference. Other factors that may have influenced the findings are the length of treatment and the doses of drugs used. Mittmann *et al.* (1997) point out that the studies included have significant heterogeneity, and these factors are among some of the differences. Different dosing regimes and efficacy of agents may also influence the lack of differences in tolerability or drop-out rate with the various drugs. On the present evidence, however, there does not appear to be support for the belief that SSRIs have fewer adverse events. The lower rates of adverse events seen in the atypical antidepressants may reflect lower doses, this may also explain the poorer efficacy.

In clinical practice treatment of depressed patients is not abandoned after a trial of one treatment. Usually further trials of antidepressants are given, sometimes in combination with other drugs, or patients are given a course of electroconvulsive therapy (ECT). It is important to consider what is the outcome of sequential treatments for a single episode of depression. Flint and Rifat (1996) attempted to address this question. They evaluated the responses of 101 elderly patients with major depression to sequential regimens of antidepressants and, if no response to drugs, a course of ECT. The protocol allowed for up to 28 weeks of treatment, initial treatment with nortriptyline that was augmented with lithium if response was poor. Non-responders were then treated with phenelzine that was augmented with lithium if there was inadequate response after 6 weeks. Finally the remaining non-responders were treated with fluoxetine (again with the potential for lithium augmentation). Patients who did not respond to pharmacotherapy were then treated with ECT; this was only discontinued if there was no response after 12 treatments. Using an intention-to-treat analysis, 83% of patients had recovered with one of the regimens by the end of the study period. For those patients who completed the protocol the outcome was very good with 94% responding to treatment. The study does illustrate that remission can be achieved in a substantial proportion of cases, although the findings may have been subject to some bias as the outcome assessments were not conducted blindly. Many clinicians would not use mono-amine oxidase inhibitors as a second-line treatment with the increasing number of different classes of antidepressants now available. Nevertheless, the reader could reasonably conclude that a treatment protocol covering a broad range of different physical treatment strategies could result in the improvement of the majority of patients with major late life depression. This view is supported by Simpson *et al.* (1998) who, in a study investigating the relationship between subtle brain changes and outcome, treated patients for 24 weeks using a broad protocol. The protocol comprised 6–12 weeks of treatment with a single antidepressant, this was followed by lithium augmentation or ECT. The overall response to this treatment was 80%.

Lithium augmentation, used in both of the above studies, has had little evaluation. Studies in elderly patients report response rates of around 25%. However, to date there have been no placebo-controlled studies and although lithium augmentation remains a strategy for resistant cases, its true value is uncertain.

In Flint and Rifat's study only a handful of patients received ECT but the outcome of depression after a course of ECT warrants consideration in its own right. ECT is widely accepted as being an effective treatment for depressive illness, possibly with a higher short-term efficacy than antidepressants. There have been very few studies of its use in depressed elderly people. Most studies report small numbers although Godber *et al.* (1987) traced the outcome of 163 patients who received ECT in a single year at an inpatient unit. Most of their cohort had previously been treated unsuccessfully with antidepressants and continued to take drugs during the course of ECT. Ninety five per cent of patients received unilateral ECT with a mean number of treatments of 11.2. The immediate outcome, not assessed by any recognized criteria, was 'fully recovered' 51% and 'much improved' 23%. The short-term efficacy of ECT is illustrated by their finding that nearly 40% of the sample had relapsed within 6 months. Whilst this study supports the efficacy of ECT in late life depression, and suggests that it may be more effective than antidepressants (74% showing substantial improvement), the reader should be aware that the study was retrospective in case selection and had other methodological flaws. However, in the absence of better evidence it is reasonable to assume that ECT has an important place in the short-term treatment of late life depression.

Longer-term outcome

The vast majority of studies into the longer-term outcome are of patients referred to psychiatric services. There have been a disproportionately large number of reports during the last two decades. Most followed a study by Murphy (1983) which painted a gloomy picture for the outcome of depression in old age. Cole (1990) and colleagues (Cole *et al.* 1997a) reviewed the literature on prognosis and conducted a meta-analysis of outcome studies. The second review included quality assessments of the studies that met the inclusion criteria. Studies were selected by searching three databases, bibliographies of retrieved articles were then searched by hand. Inclusion criteria demanded that studies had at least 20 subjects, all subjects had to be aged over 60 years, followed up for at least 1 year and assessed using affective status as outcome. Sixteen hospital based and five community studies met the inclusion criteria, involving 1487 and 249 patients, respectively. The authors found that most studies had serious methodological flaws and this point is worthy of discussion in more depth so that the reader can understand the limitations of the evidence currently available. Six aspects of quality were considered: formation of an inception cohort, description of referral pattern, completion of follow up, development and use of objective outcome criteria, blind outcome assessment, and adjustment for extraneous prognostic factors.

The formation of an inception cohort is important in that patients should be at an early and uniform point in the course of the disorder. Patients with multiple relapses or a chronic course of the depression make the prognosis appear worse than it actually is. Ideally we should study only elderly patients experiencing their first episode of depression but no studies have been this restrictive. Of the hospital-based studies the cohort studied by Murphy (1983) came closest in that subjects were over 65 years and the episode was the first one after the age of 60 – all subjects were experiencing their first episode of depression in old age but not necessarily in their lifetime. In the other studies up to 65% of the cohort had a previous history of depressive episodes.

Sample bias can also come from the referral pattern to the service. If only problem cases or unusual/interesting cases are referred then the prognosis may appear worse than it is. Similarly, if the referral process is the product of a filter system then this will have a negative effect on the outcome. This type of bias may have a large effect since less than 10% of depressed elderly patients get referred to psychiatric services (Cole and Yaffe 1996). Only three of the hospital-based studies gave some information regarding referral pattern, but this was judged to be inadequate.

Completion of follow up is crucial to any outcome study. Ideally all of the cohort should be accounted for, and a loss of more than 20% of the cohort makes any result meaningless. Two of the hospital-based studies failed to achieve this level of follow up. The outcome measures should be defined in an objective manner, together with an assurance that the outcome measures were applied in a reliable manner. All of the studies selected by Cole and Bellavance (1997a) reported outcomes in one of a number of described categories, but only three studies specified criteria for assigning subjects to these categories. A frequently used category is that of 'relapsed' but this does not distinguish between those that have short infrequent relapses and those that have a more prolonged relapse. Blind outcome assessments are particularly important if different treatments are being compared or potential prognostic indicators are being explored. Prior knowledge of clinical features or the previous course of the illness can influence outcome assessments. None of the studies included had blind outcome assessments. Lastly there should be some consideration of extraneous prognostic factors. These would include the treatments given, presence of physical disability or illness, cognitive impairment, premorbid personality and social/environmental factors. None of the studies accounted for all of these, but some studies did explore the relationship to some of these factors. Significantly, no study controlled for the treatments given or related the treatment adequacy to the prognosis.

Generally the five community-based studies included by Cole and Bellavance (1997a) were better methodologically, but sample sizes were small and all extraneous prognostic factors were not accounted for or eliminated.

Despite the methodological flaws described above together with a lack of homogeneity between the included studies, the authors carried out analyses on data pooled from the studies. The results of these analyses are described for the hospital-based and community studies separately, and for studies of less than 2 years' duration and studies of more than 2 years' duration. The results are summarized in Table 3.4.

For the hospital-based studies the average follow up in the shorter studies was 13 months, at this point almost a half of the patients had remained well. The longer studies (mean follow-up period of 52 months) had a smaller proportion of patients remaining well (27%). The combined results of both longer and shorter studies suggest that about 60% of patients have either remained well or are well but had further episodes. As already mentioned the however the chronicity or frequency of any relapses is not reported in the studies. The category of 'relapsed but recovered' should therefore be interpreted with caution as to whether this is a good outcome or not. The categories of well, relapse (with recovery), and continuously ill were consistently used in the studies. Other outcome categories such as residual symptoms, invalidism, improved, dementia, and dead are combined in Cole and Bellavance's 'Other' category.

The outcomes for the community-based studies appear to be worse both in the shorter (mean follow up 12 months) and longer (mean follow up 38 months) studies, although the wide confidence intervals reflect the smaller number of patients included in the analysis. The three studies in the longer-term analysis all reported low use of antidepressant treatment (between 4% and 33%). Under-treatment is therefore an important factor in the apparently poor prognosis of this population.

Whilst Cole and Bellavance have pointed out that the studies included were all flawed, the meta-analysis presented probably reflects the best available evidence at this time. Other criticisms of the studies include a lack of

Table 3.4. Summary of hospital- and community-based studies.

| Prognosis category | Length of follow up | | | |
| | <24 months | | >24 months | |
	Number of studies	Combined results	Number of studies	Combined results
Hospital-based studies				
Well	12	44% (36–51)	6	27% (17–38)
Recovered relapse	10	16% (14–18)	6	33% (29–36)
Continuously ill	12	22% (14–30)	5	14% (2–27)
Other	10	23% (15–30)	5	31% (21–41)
Community-based studies				
Well	2	34% (14–54)	3	19% (4–34)
Recovered relapse	–	–	–	–
Continuously ill	2	27% (6–49)	3	27% (10–44)
Other	2	31% (12–49)	3	44% (30–59)

operational diagnostic criteria and a structured interview to assess subjects in some studies, and the use of retrospective designs in others. Despite these limitations it is reasonable for the reader to conclude that the prognosis of depression in elderly people presenting to psychiatrists is better than has been suggested by some of the earlier studies. However whilst a significant proportion of patients will recover and remain well others will only achieve intermittent resolution with periods of disability which may be quite prolonged at times. In addition the reader should bear in mind that about one-third of patients will remain with unresolved symptoms or have other evidence of poor outcome.

Cole and colleagues have also reviewed the longer-term prognosis of depression in elderly community and primary care populations (Cole *et al.* 1999). Again the authors carried out a comprehensive literature search identifying over 700 potentially relevant articles. From these 12 studies met the inclusion criteria (four primary care and eight community cohorts). All studies had some methodological limitations and in those that reported the treatment received, the maximum proportion treated was 37% of the cohort. A meta-analysis was carried out and not surprisingly the combined results give a rather poor prognostic picture. At 24 month follow up 33% were well, 33% were still depressed, 21% had died, and the other 12% had other poor outcomes such as dementia or residual symptoms. The reader can conclude from this review that old age depression in community and primary care populations carries a poor prognosis, it is either chronic or relapsing or both, and is almost certainly under-treated. These results are more of a reflection of the natural course of depression in old age rather than the longer-term outcome after treatment.

The same group has also systematically reviewed the outcome of depression in medical inpatients (Cole and Bellavance 1997b). It is worth considering this patient group separately as ongoing physical disability or illness is an extraneous factor in the prognosis of depression. A thorough systematic review was carried out culminating in eight studies that met the selection criteria. These eight studies involved a total of 265 patients aged 60 years or more. A quality assessment was carried out and methodological flaws were found in all of the studies. Despite these limitations a meta-analysis was carried out. Both short-term and longer-term outcomes are reported (Table 3.5).

The outcome of this particular group of patients appears to be very poor indeed with death being a common outcome. This is far worse than the outcome of patients referred to psychiatric settings and in terms of the proportion of people recovering from depression the rate is similar to patients in community or primary care settings. Problems in detecting depression in this population and the relative lack of treatment may have a significant contribution to the poor outcome. Notably, the only study in which all of the patients were treated had the greatest rate of recovery – 39% at 1 year (Evans 1993). The mortality rate, however remained high – 48% at 1 year. Whilst the wide confidence intervals reflect imprecise results from this meta-analysis it is possible to conclude that medically ill depressed elderly patients can be successfully treated, but for those that do not recover death is a likely outcome.

Table 3.5. Summary of short- and long-term outcome studies. Figures in parentheses represent 95% confidence intervals.

Outcome	Number of studies	Combined results
Follow up less than 3 months		
Well	5	18% (6–30)
Depressed	5	43% (24–61)
Dead	3	22% (0–49)
Other	5	22% (15–28)
Follow up more than 12 months		
Well	4	19% (6–32)
Depressed	4	29% (9–50)
Dead	2	53% (18–88)
Other	4	22% (15–29)

Other vulnerable patients are those in residential and nursing homes. Ames (1990) identified 93 residents of residential care homes with significant depressive symptoms. A range of interventions, many of a social nature, was suggested by the local psychogeriatric team, but the outcome at 3 months was poor. There was no evidence of efficacy, probably because many of the suggestions had not been acted upon. At 12 months, of those who had survived, a quarter remained depressed. More recently Llewellyn-Jones *et al.* (1999) carried out a randomized control trial of a multifaceted intervention for late life depression in residential care. The intervention group had a significantly better outcome after 9 months. The average improvement on the geriatric depression scale however was modest (less than 2 points) and only 33% of the intervention group were classified as non-depressed at the endpoint and 11% of the sample had died.

Comparative outcome

So far we have considered the elderly in isolation, but does depression in old age carry a different prognosis to depression occurring at an earlier age. Studies of younger patients have found that 30% remain chronically depressed at 1–year follow up (Keller *et al.* 1992). Recently Alexopoulos et al. (1996) compared a cohort of elderly depressed patients (mean age 75 years) with a younger cohort (mean age 55 years); both groups were studied under naturalistic treatment conditions. Using survival analysis the authors found that the recovery rate for the elderly group was similar to that of the younger patients (59% and 74% probability of recovery, respectively). Within the elderly group the authors were able to compare the rate of recovery for those with their first episode in late life with those who had episodes before the age of 64 years. Late age of onset strongly predicted a slower rate of recovery. This study involved relatively small numbers and firm conclusions should not be drawn without further research. Other studies such as Meats *et al.* (1991) who compared 56 elderly patients with major depression with 24 inpatients under the age of 65. The 1–year outcome showed a significantly better prognosis for the elderly group, 68% of elderly patients were well compared with 50% of the younger patients. It is therefore reasonable to assert that old age depression does not have a worse response to treatment when compared with depression at a younger age and that depressive illness is prone to relapse, recurrence and chronicity, and this is true irrespective of age.

Other outcomes

Mortality

Although various authors have argued for and against a pessimistic outcome for old age depression, this disagreement has been limited to whether or not patients recover. Rates for mortality have been more widely agreed, and have been regarded as higher than for non-depressed elderly people. This is illustrated in Table 3.6 which shows results from both short-term and longer-term studies. A 5% year-on-year mortality is generally expected in this group, all of the studies cited have mortality rates in excess of this.

The high mortality rate (usually at least a two-fold increase) appears to be due to cardiovascular causes (Murphy *et al.* 1988, Burvill and Hall 1994). One explanation for the finding is that the depressed patients may have more pre-existing physical disease. The study by Murphy *et al.* (1988) compared two groups matched for physical morbidity as well as age and sex. The depressed group still had a statistically higher mortality. Most deaths occur early in the course of illness (Baldwin and Jolley 1986). Robinson (1989) followed up psychiatric patients for 15 years, the 2–year mortality was high at 35%, but the 10– and 15–year mortality was similar to that from the catchment population.

Other possible mechanisms for the increased mortality in depression are occult illness, illness effects (e.g. related to psychomotor retardation), treatment effects, biological effects such as abnormality of the hypothalamic–pituitary–adrenal axis or endocrine abnormalities, and suicide. Studies that have reported cause of death have found that suicides comprise a very small percentage of deaths. In order to analyse the relative mortality of elderly people

Table 3.6. Studies of mortality in depression in old age.

Author	Number	Follow up (months)	Mortality rate (%)
Murphy 1983	124	12	14
Rabins et al. 1985	62	12	13
Burvill et al. 1991	103	12	11
Baldwin et al. 1993	98	12	19
Murphy et al.	120	48	34
Baldwin and Jolley 1986	100	48	26

with depression Pulska *et al.* (1998) carried out a survival analysis of 29 elderly depressed patients and 853 control subjects followed up for 6 years. The results support a higher risk of mortality in the depressed subjects – relative risk 2.0 (95% CI 1.17–3.41).

Higher mortality has also been found in community samples and in depressed medical inpatients. In the latter group it may be that active antidepressant treatment does not improve the mortality rate. In a small study of 23 depressed medical inpatients, Evans (1993) found that the 1–year mortality was 48% despite all patients receiving antidepressant treatment.

Dementia

A number of studies have found that late life depression is not associated with an increased risk of dementia (Murphy 1983, Baldwin and Jolley 1986, Stoudemire *et al.* 1993). The presence of depressive pseudodementia, however, may have some association with future cognitive impairment. Alexopoulos *et al.* (1993) studied 57 depressed inpatients subdivided by the presence or not of 'reversible dementia'. Using survival analysis, there was an almost five-fold increase in the risk of developing dementia, but it is possible that some of those studied were already demented at presentation, even though their cognitive function improved temporarily with treatment. This was a relatively small study and firm conclusions should not be drawn, but we should be aware that depressive pseudodementia may be a prodrome of a dementia.

Factors predicting outcome

Various factors that may predict or influence the prognosis of late life depression have been suggested and studied. These include the presence of cognitive impairment, physical ill health, first episode before the age of 60 years, advanced age at onset, severity of depressive symptoms including presence of psychotic symptoms, presence of previous episodes, marital status, and living circumstances. In addition the presence of intervening life events, social class, presence of major social difficulties, presence of confiding relationships, and premorbid personality traits have been studied. Lastly, the presence of both coarse brain disease and more subtle cerebral changes have been considered.

Cole and Bellavance (1997a) in their systematic review of the prognosis considered the factors that had been considered in their selected studies. As already mentioned they had detected significant heterogeneity between these studies, in addition they found that there was a great variation in the definition and measurement of factors between studies. As a consequence they were unable to carry out a meta-analysis on the data relating to prognostic factors. This is unfortunate as many of the studies were of insufficient size in order to have the power to detect an association between factor and outcome. The authors did however summarize the effect of the various factors reported in the studies. Six studies reported the effect of cognitive impairment, three of them associating poor outcome with cognitive impairment. Physical ill health was associated with poor outcome in six out of 10 studies. Age of onset of the first depressive episode was linked with poor prognosis in three studies but not in four others. Advanced age predicted poor outcome in two out of five studies. Four studies found that the severity of depressive symptoms was linked to poor outcome, but five others refuted this. Previous episodes were predictive of poor prognosis in two out of three studies.

A number of studies considered the effect of social factors. Seven reported that marital status and living circumstances were not related to the prognosis, but one reported that living alone was linked to a poor outcome. Property ownership was related to a good outcome in one study. Severe intervening life events predicted a poor outcome in two studies, but were associated with good outcome in a third. One study considered the effects of social class, major social difficulties, and the presence of a confiding relationship; an association with outcome was not found. Another study looked at employment, social contact, income, and changes in living circumstances and concluded that favourable social circumstances were linked with a better outcome. The presence of abnormal personality traits was associated with poor outcome in one out of three studies.

It is clear from the above that there is conflicting and inconsistent evidence regarding the role of the above factors in the outcome of late life depression. Clearly some of the factors lend themselves to intervention, for example ongoing physical ill health or social difficulties. It seems obvious that interventions to improve these will probably lead to an improved quality of life for the patient even if the prognosis of the depressive episode is not altered in the long run. As for the factors that cannot be altered by interventions then their presence may suggest a more aggressive treatment approach at an earlier stage. However, in the absence of conclusive evidence about their role the clinician should be aware that over-treatment may burden the patient with unnecessary side-effects from medication. On the other hand, if tolerance to treatment is well established it would seem unwise to discontinue prophylactic medication in the presence of intervening life events or other factors.

Most of the studies selected by Cole and Bellavance (1997a) had excluded patients with significant cognitive impairment. The tendency to exclude patients with dementia or structural brain damage in these studies is understandable. In a clinical setting, however, it is not uncommon for patients to have depression and co-existing brain disease. Baldwin et al. (1993) compared the outcome of 32 depressed patients who also had coarse cerebral disease (dementia or stroke) with 66 depressed patients without such co-morbidity. Unfortunately the two groups were not ideally matched. At 1–year follow up the co-morbid group had a poorer outcome but this was not statistically significant. The co-morbid group had a greater mortality and this largely accounts for the poorer outcome. However, more studies are required before we can conclude one way or another about the effects of coarse brain disease on the prognosis. This study does suggest that treatment of depression in the presence of co-morbidity can be successful.

Subtle cerebral changes as evidenced on psychometric testing or by neuro-imaging have been linked to depression in late life. Several studies have explored the association between these changes and the outcome of the depression. Beats *et al.* (1996) studied frontal lobe function in 24 elderly depressed patients and 15 matched controls. Higher residual depression scores were associated with slowed thinking times and increased ventricular size. Simpson *et al.* (1998) studied 75 patients whose response to treatment was classified as good, partial resistance, and absolute resistance. Magnetic resonance imaging (MRI) was performed on 44 of the patients, 66 of the patients had detailed neuropsychological testing. Evidence of deep white matter hyperintensities was significantly greater in the resistant patients. The psychometric test abnormalities that were associated with treatment resistance were tests that reflect frontal or subcortical function. O'Brien *et al.* (1998) studied 54 depressed patients aged 55 years or over. Twenty-five per cent had severe white matter lesions present on MRI scanning, after a mean follow up of 32 months these patients had a significantly worse outcome. A survival analysis showed a median survival (to relapse) of 136 days in those with severe lesions compared with 315 days in those without. Unfortunately, the treatment given to the subjects is not described in the study. All of these studies support the notion that subtle cerebral changes are related to treatment response in late life depression. It may therefore be worth taking into account such findings when considering the length of specialist monitoring and the use of prophylactic antidepressants.

Improving the prognosis

There is certainly room for improvement in the prognosis of late life depression. A significant proportion of elderly depressed patients does not achieve a full remission. At least a third will not respond to treatment with a single antidepressant. Which treatment strategy should follow this is open to debate but the limited evidence does suggest that vigorous treatment with antidepressants and/or ECT is associated with a better outcome. Although a persistent and aggressive treatment strategy seems obvious the community-based studies of outcome suggest that under-treatment is so prevalent that no treatment at all is the norm. Likewise in the naturalistic cohort studies describing prognosis at 1 year and beyond there is also evidence of under-treatment, in particular the use of ECT is very variable yet this treatment may be the most effective in the short-term. The reader should also bear in mind that even when treatment is prescribed this may be at a sub-therapeutic level, using antidepressant assays to assess dosing adequacy Jerling (1995) found that tricyclic antidepressants were often used in sub-optimal doses.

When faced with a patient whose depression does not show significant improvement after 6 weeks the following options should be considered. Firstly, extend the trial beyond the 'traditional' 6–week period, ensuring the dose is optimal. A further trial of 6 weeks may be beneficial but if the patient is distressed or deteriorating other options should be considered. Secondly, change to an antidepressant of another class, this is a popular and logical strategy for which there is surprisingly little evidence. Thirdly, use augmentation strategy or combine different classes of antidepressants. Fourthly, consider a course of ECT.

Once achieving remission the clinician must consider continuation therapy to reduce the risk of relapse, and consider longer-term prophylaxis. In general adult psychiatry the period after remission carrying a high risk of relapse is usually regarded as 6 months. In the elderly this period may be longer, perhaps up to 2 years. An optimal length of continuation therapy has never been established but the UK Old Age Depression Interest Group (OADIG) study found that most relapses occurred in the first 12 months (OADIG 1993), and this may represent a reasonable minimum period for continuation therapy.

With regard to longer-term prophylaxis the OADIG (1993) study entered 69 patients who recovered sufficiently to a 2–year double-blind placebo-controlled trial of dothiepin. Survival analysis showed that dothiepin (75 mg daily) significantly reduced the risk of relapse/recurrence. However, 30% of those in the actively treated group still experienced a relapse, so there is scope for further improvement. This finding together with the generally high rate of recurrence and relapse in late life depression supports the argument for indefinite prophylactic treatment. Given that the life expectancy of a patient in their seventies is on average 5 years then the gain from preventing 6 months morbidity due to a recurrence of depressive illness becomes significant. Against this argument are the potential side-effects from long-term drug use, particularly weight gain. These problems may be less marked with newer antidepressants although the short-term data on adverse events would suggest there is little difference between older and newer agents (Mittmann *et al.* 1997). Also against the argument for indefinite prophylaxis is the fact that a noticeable proportion of the placebo group remained well during the study period. Prophylactic treatment of these patients would potentially have burdened the patient with unwanted drug side-effects without any health gain. Unfortunately, reliably identifying those who are at risk remains elusive although those with two or more recurrences in the past 2 years, serious ill health, chronic social difficulties or very severe depression at the outset are most likely to be at risk given our current knowledge.

Key points

- Untreated depression in old age has a poor prognosis with chronicity and high mortality.
- Two-thirds of patients will significantly improve with pharmacological treatment.
- In the long term, less than half of those treated will remain well; relapse, chronicity and other outcomes are common.
- Depressed medical inpatients have a very poor prognosis.
- There is a two-fold increased risk of death associated with late life depression.

References

Alexopoulos, G.S., Meyers, B.S., Young, R.C., Mattis, S. and Kakuma, T. (1993) The course of geriatric depression with 'reversible dementia': a controlled study. *American Journal of Psychiatry*, **150**, 1693–1699.

Alexopoulos, G.S., Meyers, B.S., Young, R.C., Kakuma, T., Feder, M., Einhorn, A. *et al.* (1996) Recovery in geriatric depression. *Archives of General Psychiatry*, **53**, 305–312.

Ames, D. (1990) Depression among elderly residents of local-authority residential homes. *British Journal of Psychiatry*, **156**, 667–675.

Baldwin, R.C. (1991) The outcome of depression in old age. *International Journal of Geriatric Psychiatry*, **6**, 395–400.

Baldwin, R.C. and Jolley, D.J. (1986) The prognosis of depression in old age. *British Journal of Psychiatry*, **149**, 574–583.

Baldwin, R.C., Benbow, S.M., Marriott, A. and Tomenson, B. (1993) The prognosis of depression in later life: a reconsideration of cerebral organic factors in relation to outcome. *British Journal of Psychiatry*, **163**, 82–90.

Beats, B.C., Sahakian, B.J. and Levy, R. (1996) Cognitive performance in tests sensitive to frontal lobe dysfunction in the elderly depressed. *Psychological Medicine*, **26**, 591–603.

Burvill, P. W., Hall, W.D., Stampfer, H.G., and Emmerson, J.P. (1991) The prognosis of depression in old age. *British Journal of Psychiatry*, **158**, 64–71.

Burvill, P. W. and Hall, W.D. (1994) Predictors of increased mortality in elderly depressed patients. *International Journal of Geriatric Psychiatry*, **9**, 219–227.

Cole, M.G. (1990) The prognosis of depression in the elderly. *Canadian Medical Association Journal*, **143**, 633–640.

Cole, M.G. and Yaffe, M.J. (1996) Pathway to psychiatric care of the elderly with depression. *International Journal of Geriatric Psychiatry*, **11**, 157–161.

Cole, M.G. and Bellavance, F. (1997a) The prognosis of depression in old age. *American Journal of Geriatric Psychiatry*, **5**, 4–14.

Cole, M.G. and Bellavance, F. (1997b) Depression in elderly medical inpatients: a meta-analysis of outcomes. *Canadian Medical Association Journal*, **157**, 1055–1060.

Cole, M.G., Bellavance, F., and Mansour, A. (1999) Prognosis of depression in elderly community and primary care populations: a systematic review and meta-analysis. *American Journal of Psychiatry*, **156**, 1182–1189.

Evans, M.E. (1993) Depression in elderly physically ill in-patients: a 12 month prospective study. *International Journal of Geriatric Psychiatry*, **8**, 587–592.

Flint, A.J. and Rifat, S.L. (1996) The effect of sequential antidepressant treatment on geriatric depression. *Journal of Affective Disorders*, **36**, 95–105.

Godber, C., Rosenvinge, H., Wilkinson, D., and Smithies, J. (1987) Depression in old age: prognosis after ECT. *International Journal of Geriatric Psychiatry*, **2**, 19–24.

Jerling, M. (1995) Dosing of antidepressants – the unknown art. *Journal of Clinical Psychopharmacology*, **15**, 435–439.

Keller, M.B., Lavori, P. V., Mueller, T.I., Endicott, J., Coryell, W., Hirschfeldt *et al.* (1992) Time to recovery, chronicity, and levels of psychochpathology in major depression. *Archives of General Psychiatry*, **49**, 809–816.

Llewellyn-Jones, R.H., Baikie, K.A., Smithers, H., Cohen, J., Snowden J. and Tennent, C.C. (1999) Multifaceted shared care intervention for late life depression in residential care: randomised control trial. *British Medical Journal*, **319**, 676–681.

McCusker, J., Cole, M., Keller, E., Bellavance, F., and Berard, A. (1998) Effectiveness of treatments of depression in older ambulatory patients. *Archives of Internal Medicine*, **158**, 705–712.

Meats, P. , Timol, M., and Jolley, D. (1991) Prognosis of depression in the elderly. *British Journal of Psychiatry*, **159**, 659–663.

Mittmann, N., Herrmann, N., Einarson, T.R., Busto, U.E., Lanctot, K.L., Liu, B.A., *et al.* (1997) The efficacy, safety and tolerability of antidepressants in late life depression: a meta-analysis. *Journal of Affective Disorders*, **46**, 191–217.

Murphy, E. (1983) The prognosis of depression in old age. *British Journal of Psychiatry*, **142**, 111–119.

Murphy, E., Smith, R., Lindesay, J., and Slattery, J. (1988) Increased mortality rates in late-life depression. *British Journal of Psychiatry*, **152**, 347–353.

O'Brien, J., Ames, D., Chiu, E., Schweitzer, I., Desmond, P. , and Tress, B. (1998) Severe deep white matter lesions and outcome in elderly patients with major depressive disorder: follow up study. *British Medical Journal*, **317**, 982–984.

Old Age Depression Interest Group (1993) How long should the elderly take antidepressants? A double-blind placebo-controlled study of continuation/prophylaxis therapy with dothiepin. *British Journal of Psychiatry*, **162**, 175–182.

Pulska, T., Pahkala, K., Laippala, P. and Kivela S-L. (1998) Major depression as a predictor of premature deaths in elderly people in Finland: a community study. *Acta Psychiatrica Scandinavia*, **97**, 408–411.

Rabins, P. V., Harvis, K., and Koven S. (1985) High fatality rates of late-life depression associated with cardiovascular disease. *Journal of Affective Disorders*, **9**, 165–167.

Robinson, J.R. (1989) The natural history of mental disorder in old age: a long-term study. *British Journal of Psychiatry*, **154**, 783–789.

Sharma, V.K., Copeland, J.R.M., Dewey, M.E., Lowe, D., and Davidson, I. (1998) Outcome of the depressed elderly living in the community in Liverpool: a five year follow-up. *Psychological Medicine*, **28**, 1329–1337.

Simpson, S., Baldwin, R.C., Jackson, A., and Burns, A.S. (1998) Is sub-cortical disease associated with a poor response to antidepressants? Neurological, neuropsychological and neuroradiological findings in late-life depression. *Psychological Medicine*, **28**, 1015–1026.

Stoudemire, A., Hill, C., Morris, R., Martino-Saltzman, D., and Lewison, B. (1993) Long-term affective and cognitive outcome in depressed older adults. *American Journal of Psychiatry*, **150**, 896–900.

The pharmacological treatment of depression in older people

4

Simon Wilson and Stephen Curran

Introduction

Why is the pharmacological treatment of depression different in older people?

Which antidepressants are most effective in the elderly?

Which are the safest antidepressants in the elderly?

What is the optimum dose of antidepressants in the elderly?

How long does it take for elderly patients to respond to antidepressants?

How long should antidepressants be continued after remission?

How quickly should antidepressants be withdrawn?

What if there is no response to the first-choice antidepressant?

Introduction

This chapter discusses the pharmacological treatment of depression in older people. Although important, medication only forms part of the successful management of depression in the elderly. It is important to adopt a multi-disciplinary approach to management and consider psychological and social interventions such as bereavement counselling, occupational therapy, cognitive–behavioural psychotherapy or family therapy.

As well as taking a full history and carrying out a mental state examination, physical assessment of patients is particularly important in the elderly before embarking on pharmacological treatment. Physical illness can cause depression, e.g. hypothyroidism; affect the choice of medication, e.g. avoiding tricyclic antidepressants (TCAs) in prostatic hypertrophy; and can be an important maintaining factor, e.g. disability because of arthritis.

Why is the pharmacological treatment of depression different in older people?

Older people are more sensitive to the side-effects of drugs and experience adverse events more frequently than younger patients. Pharmacodynamic and pharmacokinetic changes with increasing age both play a part in explaining increased drug sensitivity (Lader 1994). Pharmacodynamic changes include increased receptor sensitivity and a reduction in total receptor numbers with increasing age. Changes in drug distribution, metabolism and excretion are the main pharmacokinetic factors involved. A shift in body composition with a relative reduction in total body water compared to fat alters the distribution of lipid-soluble drugs in particular. As a result, the half-life of many lipid-soluble psychotropic drugs is prolonged. Hepatic metabolism of psychotropic drugs is reduced because of decreased hepatic blood flow and slowed enzyme metabolism. Glomerular filtration rate declines by 50% between young adulthood and the age of 70 (Lader 1994), which is of particular importance in explaining the increased risk of lithium toxicity in older patients. The increased likelihood of concurrent physical illness in the elderly together with the increased likelihood of drug interactions due to polypharmacy also plays a large part in explaining increased risk of adverse events with psychotropic medication.

When prescribing an antidepressant to an older patient, it is wise to adhere to the maxim 'Start low and go slow' (Baldwin and Burns 1998). A small starting dose and a gradual increase in dose is necessary if troublesome side-effects are to be avoided. Although the elderly as a group are more sensitive to medication, there is wide inter-subject variation in drug metabolism with up to a 10–fold variation in plasma levels between patients given the same dose of antidepressant (Bertilsson and Dahl 1996). For this reason some older patients can tolerate an equivalent dose of antidepressant to that used in younger patients provided increases in dose are carried out gradually and the patient is monitored closely for side-effects.

Faced with an elderly patient suffering from depression, our task is to navigate the often narrow channel between the unpleasant and potentially hazardous side-effects of antidepressants, and the persistent morbidity, disability and risk of suicide if the depression is inadequately treated. In negotiating this channel safely the clinician has to weigh several factors in the choice of antidepressant medication. The range of antidepressants available means that treatment can, to some extent, be tailored to the individual patient to take account of symptoms, severity of depression, the presence of physical illness, patient preference and likely tolerance of side-effects. Table 4.1 lists the classes of antidepressants that can be considered as first-line treatments together with their mode of action and some characteristics when used in older patients.

Table 4.1. Classification of antidepressants.

Class	Examples	Mode of action	Characteristics
Tricyclics (TCAs)	Amitriptyline Nortriptyline Lofepramine	Alpha-1 adrenergic antagonism 5HT-2 antagonism	Potential problems with: • anticholinergic side effects; • confusion • postural hypotension • atrioventricular heart block.
Selective serotonin re-uptake inhibitors (SSRIs)	Fluoxetine Paroxetine Citalopram	Block pre-synaptic re-uptake of serotonin (5HT)	In general well tolerated in the elderly. Liquid preparations available. Gastrointestinal upset and akathisia cause problems in some.
Monoamine oxidase inhibitors (MAOIs)	Phenelzine Tranylcypramine	Irreversible inhibition of the enzyme monoamine oxidase A	Risk of hypertensive crisis with tyramine rich foods and over-the-counter sympathomimetic 'cold cures'. Postural hypotension and insomnia limit use in the elderly.
Reversible inhibitors of monoamine oxidase (RIMAs)	Moclobemide	Reversible inhibition of the enzyme monoamine oxidase A	Better tolerated in the elderly than MAOIs. Fewer dietary restrictions.
5HT-2 antagonists	Trazodone Nefazodone	Serotonin re-uptake blockade with post-synaptic 5HT-2 antagonism	Useful in the elderly as 5HT-2 antagonism reduces anxiety. Trazodone is more sedative as it also blocks histamine receptors.
Noradrenaline and serotonin re-uptake (NSRIs)	Venlafaxine	Block pre-synaptic re-uptake of noradrenaline and serotonin	At lower doses side-effects similar to SSRIs. At higher doses can cause insomnia and exacerbate hypertension.
Noradrenergic and specific serotonergic antidepressant (NaSSA)	Mirtazapine	Blocks inhibitory alpha-2 presynaptic receptors increasing noradrenaline release Increased 5HT release Blocks 5HT-2 and 5HT-3 receptors reducing unwanted side-effects	Theoretically of use in depression associated with anxiety and agitation but little evidence on which to base use in the elderly to date. Sedative at lower doses.

Which antidepressants are most effective in the elderly?

Most drug trials comparing the efficacy of antidepressants have excluded patients over the age of 65 and those with significant physical illness. This has resulted in a relative lack of evidence on which to base decisions when treating patients over the age of 65. Livingstone and Livingston (1999) have reviewed five double-blind randomized-controlled trials which have compared TCAs with newer antidepressants (SSRIs and venlafaxine) in patients over the age of 65. All five trials found that TCAs and the newer antidepressants were equally effective. However, none of the trials included enough subjects to detect small differences in efficacy and patients with significant physical illness were excluded.

Given equal efficacy, the choice of first-line antidepressants in the elderly is strongly influenced in favour of those antidepressants which are least likely to cause troublesome side-effects. However, there are some particular groups of patients where evidence can guide the choice of antidepressant. Firstly, there is evidence that TCAs are more effective than SSRIs (selective serotonin reuptake inhibitors) in treating patients with severe melancholic-type depression characterized by anhedonia, diurnal mood variation, early morning wakening and psychomotor retardation or agitation (Roose et al. 1994). Secondly, patients suffering from severe depression associated with mood-congruent delusions require a different treatment from the outset. In this group of patients, antidepressants used alone are less likely to be effective and a combination of antidepressant with an antipsychotic is usually necessary (Spiker et al. 1985). Delusional depression in the elderly seems to be more resistant to pharmacotherapy than in younger patients (Baldwin 1988) and electroconvulsive therapy (ECT) may be the treatment of choice in this group of patients (Flint and Rifat 1998).

In younger patients, the monoamine oxidase inhibitors (MAOIs) have been thought to be of particular use in depression characterized by anxiety and an absence of melancholic features. Unfortunately the traditional MAOIs can cause marked postural hypotension in the elderly and Taylor et al. (1999) have advised that they are avoided in the elderly. Moclobemide, a reversible inhibitor of monoamine oxidase (RIMA), requires little or no dietary restrictions and is well tolerated in the elderly and may be a useful alternative for depressed patients with prominent anxiety and an absence of melancholic features.

Elderly patients who have cognitive impairment complicated by depression are prone to side-effects, particularly the anticholinergic effects of TCAs, which exacerbate pre-existing confusion. Moclobemide has been shown to be of value in treating depression in elderly patients with cognitive impairment (Roth et al. 1996) and may be a first-line antidepressant in this group of patients.

Which are the safest antidepressants in the elderly?

Older TCAs (e.g. amitriptyline and imipramine) are often not chosen as first-line antidepressants in the elderly because of potentially hazardous side-effects, particularly in those patients with heart disease. Newer TCAs (e.g. lofepramine) and SSRIs are often used in preference as first line antidepressants. Table 4.2 lists the more common side-effects of TCAs and SSRIs.

Meta-analyses of the drop-out rates from trials comparing antidepressants suggest that SSRIs are better tolerated than the older TCAs with 10% fewer patients being withdrawn from trials (Anderson and Tomerson 1995). However, this does not seem to be the case for trials in which SSRIs were compared with newer TCAs or heterocyclic antidepressants (e.g. Trazodone) where there was no difference in the rates of patients withdrawn from treatment (Song *et al*. 1993). These findings have been confirmed in a more recent meta-analysis of patients withdrawn from trials by Hoptopf *et al*. (1997). The importance of this study is that Hoptopf *et al*. went on to examine 11 trials that included elderly patients and found that drop-out rates did not differ significantly from younger patients.

One of the difficulties in interpreting the clinical significance of drop-out rates from randomized-controlled trials of antidepressants is that drop-out rates alone give no indication of the seriousness of events which led to

Table 4.2. Common and important side-effects of TCAs and SSRIs.

Tricyclic antidepressants	SSRIs
Alpha-1 adrenergic receptor blockade:	**5HT-3 receptor stimulation:**
Postural hypotension	Nausea
Dizziness	Headache
	Gastrointestinal upset
Muscarinic receptor blockade:	**5HT-2 receptor stimulation:**
Constipation	Agitation
Blurred vision	Akathisia
Dry mouth	Insomnia
Urinary retention	Sexual dysfunction
Delirium	
Tachycardia	
Heart block	
Histamine receptor blockade:	
Weight gain	
Drowsiness	
Hyponatraemia:	
More common in the elderly. Presents with vague symptoms which may be attributed to depression, e.g. lassitude and headaches.	

antidepressants being withdrawn. For example, one group of patients may have had antidepressants withdrawn because of nausea while another group experienced falls and postural hypotension, with potentially far greater consequences. When comparing SSRIs with older antidepressants, it should be remembered that SSRIs are not without troublesome and potentially hazardous side-effects in the elderly, e.g. hyponatraemia (Table 4.2).

A further reason for favouring SSRIs as first-line antidepressants over the older TCAs in the elderly is toxicity in overdose. The risk results from the propensity of the older TCAs to cause cardiac arrhythmias or seizures at toxic levels (Edwards 1995). Dothiepin, seems to be particularly risky in overdose (Buckley *et al.* 1994). In comparison, the SSRIs are safer, with fewer adverse events reported after overdose (Case History 4.1).

Case History 4.1

A 75–year-old man was admitted to hospital with an exacerbation of chronic obstructive airways disease. He had become more anxious and worried about his health since the sudden death of a friend 3 months before. He had been commenced on dothiepin by his GP because of tearfulness and sleep disturbance. While on the medical ward he had periods of confusion at night and complained of difficulty passing urine. On examination he was anxious and preoccupied with his physical health. Orientation at the time of the examination was normal. A diagnosis of a depressive episode was made. His nocturnal confusion was thought to be secondary to a combination of hypoxia and the anticholinergic effects of dothiepin which was also causing prostatism. The dothiepin was discontinued and paroxetine commenced. He had no further episodes of confusion and his mood had returned to normal when seen 4 weeks later.

What is the optimum dose of antidepressants in the elderly?

The elderly are more sensitive to the side-effects of antidepressants than younger patients (Lader 1994). It is important to start with lower doses of antidepressants in the elderly and increase gradually. Smaller than standard doses of antidepressants may be effective in the elderly. However, there is wide inter-subject variation in drug metabolism and some elderly patients may require and tolerate doses of antidepressants equivalent to those used in younger patients provided the dose is increased gradually.

Where patients are sensitive to TCAs at relatively low doses nortriptyline could be used with monitoring of plasma levels. Therapeutic plasma concentrations have been determined for nortriptyline and it is well-tolerated in elderly patients and those with cardiovascular disease (Roose *et al.* 1994).

How long does it take for elderly patients to respond to antidepressants?

In about one-third of patients there will be an inadequate response to the first antidepressant used (Flint 1985). How long should one wait for a response? In younger patients a 4–week trial of antidepressant is generally considered adequate with a change to a different class of antidepressant if there is no response (Spigset and Martensson 1999). Quitken *et al.* (1984) have shown that improvement can be delayed to between 4 and 6 weeks and a trial of 8 weeks may be necessary for a response to occur in the elderly (Georgotas and McCue 1989). The likelihood of obtaining a response by extending the use of an antidepressant beyond 4 weeks has to be weighed against the distress and risks of persistent depression for each patient. It may be necessary to give ECT if the response to antidepressants is delayed or slow and there is a concern about suicide risk. If there has been no response after 4 weeks the antidepressant should be changed to a different class or ECT considered. If there has been a partial response at 4 weeks the antidepressant can be continued with regular monitoring of the mental state to ensure that the improvement continues. If there is evidence of a high suicide risk, psychotic depression or marked psychomotor agitation or retardation then ECT should be considered (Case History 4.2).

Case History 4.2

A 77 year old woman was referred by her GP after investigations in hospital for nausea and vomiting had failed to reveal a cause. While in hospital she had been seen by a psychiatrist and commenced on fluoxetine 20 mg daily. She continued to experience anorexia and nausea on returning home and had lost weight. On examination she was agitated and distressed. She explained that she could not eat because food would stick in her throat. She frequently checked her mouth by looking in a mirror. She was admitted urgently to hospital with a diagnosis of a severe depressive episode with possible hypochondriacal delusions. The fluoxetine was stopped and she was commenced on doxepin which was increased to 150 mg daily. She remained distressed but improved markedly after five treatments of ECT. She remained well on doxepin 150 mg 2 years later.

How long should antidepressants be continued after remission?

The elderly are at a high risk of recurrence following a depressive episode, with up to a 70% risk of recurrence within 2 years of remission (Flint 1992). Continuation treatment for 6 months after full remission is now standard practice in patients under 65 years of age. Flint (1992) cites evidence to support using continuation treatment beyond 6 months in the elderly. Firstly, naturalistic studies of untreated depression in the elderly suggest a duration of 12–48 months. Secondly, the risk of recurrence after a single depressive episode in the elderly is high and about the same as that for younger patients with a history of recurrent depression. Lastly, with further episodes, there is a tendency to shorter periods of remission, longer duration of episodes and increasing treatment resistance.

One of the few placebo-controlled trials of maintenance antidepressants in patients over the age of 65 showed that dothiepin 75 mg daily reduced the relative risk of recurrence by a factor of 2.5 (Old Age Depression Interest Group 1993). As there are few trials of maintenance treatment in the elderly the results from trials in younger patients may provide some general guidance:

- The antidepressant which led to remission is likely to be equally effective in continuation or maintenance treatment.
- The dose of antidepressant which led to remission is likely to be the most effective at continuing remission and preventing relapse (Frank *et al.* 1990).
- Given the high risk of recurrence within 2 years of a first depressive episode after the age of 60, continuation treatment should be for at least 1 year, and probably 2 (Prien and Kupfer 1986).

Given these factors, there is a strong argument for long-term maintenance pharmacotherapy in the elderly beyond 2 years.

How quickly should antidepressants be withdrawn?

A discontinuation syndrome has been described for most antidepressants, especially following abrupt withdrawal. Symptoms experienced by patients who have abruptly stopped antidepressants are listed in Table 4.3. To avoid a discontinuation syndrome, continuation or maintenance antidepressants taken for longer than 1 year should be withdrawn over 6–8 weeks, and possibly more slowly if taken as maintenance for several years. Withdrawal of antidepressants over 1 week is probably adequate for courses lasting less than 8 weeks (Drug and Therapeutics Bulletin 1999).

A discontinuation syndrome can occur in up to 50% of patients suddenly withdrawing from tricyclic antidepressants (Drug and Therapeutics Bulletin 1999). Of the SSRIs paroxetine seems to be at particular risk of leading to a discontinuation syndrome, probably because of its shorter half-life. Discontinuation symptoms usually start abruptly and resolve within 24 h if the antidepressant is re-started. The discontinuation syndrome can usually be distinguished from the early recurrence of depression. Recurrence of depression is rare within 1 week of stopping antidepressants and resolves more slowly than the discontinuation syndrome after antidepressants are re-started (Case History 4.3).

Table 4.3. Symptoms of the antidepressant discontinuation syndrome (Drugs and Therapeutics Bulletin 1999).

- Fatigue
- Insomnia
- Anxiety
- Nightmares
- Sweating
- Tremor
- Nausea
- Parasthesiae
- Headache
- Poor balance

Case History 4.3

A 66–year-old woman was referred urgently by her GP with a recent worsening of anxiety. She had a history of recurrent depression and had been maintained on amitriptyline for a number of years until changed to paroxetine 1 year before when she experienced palpitations. Her GP suspected an agitated depression. When seen she complained of insomnia, headaches and parasthesiae. She described increased anxiety and palpitations since a friend was robbed in the street 1 week before. She had stopped the paroxetine 2 days before fearing that this was causing the palpitations. A diagnosis of SSRI discontinuation syndrome was made. She was advised to recommence the paroxetine and she was reviewed the following day when most of her symptoms had resolved. She was referred to a day hospital for anxiety management.

What if there is no response to the first-choice antidepressant?

Given that 30–40% of patients will fail to respond to an initial antidepressant, this is a common clinical scenario (Flint 1995). At this stage patients may be discouraged and so clinicians should maintain a positive outlook and reassure the patient that this is not unusual. Before considering any changes in pharmacotherapy it is important to review the diagnosis, ask whether medication has been taken and address psychosocial factors which may be maintaining the depression. A list of factors to consider before making changes to pharmacotherapy is given in Table 4.4. Once these factors have been addressed changes to pharmacotherapy can be pursued.

The following sections examine the treatment options when there is no response to a first-choice antidepressant.

(a) Increase the dose of antidepressant

This is a useful option in younger patients with up to 50% of patients with refractory depression responding in one study (Bridges *et al*. 1995). However,

Table 4.4. Factors to consider if there is no response to an antidepressant

Is there another relevant diagnosis?

- Organic mood disorder: physical examination, blood screen, chest X-ray.
- Psychotic depression: repeat mental state examination.
- 'Vascular depression': history of cerebrovascular disease, associated with slow response to antidepressants (Alexopoulos et al. 1997).
- Harmful use of alcohol or dependence: CAGE questionnaire, MCV, γGT.

Has the antidepressant been taken?

- Ask about side-effects and concerns.
- Patient may not have returned to GP for repeat prescription.
- Patient may not wish to volunteer side-effects, particularly sexual dysfunction.
- Fear of becoming 'addicted'.

Are social or family problems maintaining the depressed mood?

- Social isolation: refer to day centre or day hospital.
- Recent bereavement or loss.
- Poverty, with inadequate housing or diet: refer to Social Services.
- Marital discord.
- High expressed emotion in relatives.
- Difficult family life-cylce transition.
- Consider referral to CPN for marital/family work.

decreased tolerance of higher doses limits its usefulness in the elderly. Some older patients may be able to tolerate a gradual increase in dose of a TCA with regular monitoring for side-effects and measurement of lying and standing blood pressure. There is little evidence that increasing doses of SSRIs improves outcome (Baldwin 1999).

(b) Change to a different class of antidepressant

In most cases the choice will involve switching from an SSRI to TCA or vice versa although newer antidepressants have increased the therapeutic options. There is little evidence that switching within classes of antidepressants is of benefit (Baldwin 1999).

Wattis et al. (1994) surveyed the use of antidepressants by psychiatrists working with the elderly. Lofepramine and dothiepin were the most commonly prescribed antidepressants. Of the SSRIs, fluoxetine was most commonly used. Other commonly used antidepressants were amitriptyline, trazodone, clomipramine and doxepin. It is perhaps surprising that dothiepin and amitriptyline were commonly used, despite their propensity to cause side-effects. However, the survey was undertaken before many of the new antidepressants were available.

(c) Use of ECT

It should be borne in mind when treating depression in the elderly that switching from one antidepressant to another involves delay as it takes time to increase doses to therapeutic levels. ECT should be considered at any point in treatment but particularly when there are psychotic symptoms, severe psychomotor agitation or retardation or risk of death from self-neglect or suicide.

There are important interactions between pharmacotherapy and ECT and these are summarized in Table 4.5.

(d) Augmentation

If there has been no or only partial response to two antidepressants from different classes, augmentation should be considered. A number of augmentation strategies have been advocated, including use of lithium, tri-iodothyronine, anti-epileptic drugs and antidepressant combinations.

Table 4.5. Drug interactions with ECT (Curran and Freeman 1995)

Benzodiazepines	Reduced effectiveness of ECT. Raise seizure threshold and decrease seizure duration so more treatments are needed.
	Long-established benzodiazepines should not be stopped suddenly before ECT.
Tricyclic antidepressants	Little evidence of effect on seizure threshold during ECT.
Selective serotonin re-uptake inhibitors (SSRIs)	Prolonged seizures reported. Start with low initial treatment stimulus.
Monoamine oxidase inhibitors (MAOIs)	Increased seizure threshold may lead to shorter seizures. Do not need to be stopped before ECT but the anaethetist should be aware that the patient is taking an MAOI.
Lithium	Reduces seizure threshold. More severe memory impairment reported, which may be related to lower fit threshold and excess electrical stimulus.
	Start with low stimulus dose and monitor cognitive function.
Anticonvulsants	Raise seizure threshold and decreased seizure duration.
	Continue anticonvulsants during ECT but high stimulus doses may be required when anticonvulsants are used for mood disorders.
Antipsychotics	In general lower seizure threshold.
	The manufacturers recommend suspending Clozapine for 24 hours before ECT.

Evidence for the efficacy of augmentation mainly comes from studies in younger patients. The few studies that have included elderly patients have used lithium augmentation (see review by Flint 1995). In a survey of patients over 65 years of age who were prescribed lithium, Head and Denning (1998) found that 38% were prescribed lithium for a depressive illness. Prospective controlled trials of lithium use in the elderly have reported response rates of about 20% (Flint and Rifat 1994), which is less than the response rate in younger patients of about 35% (Baldwin 1999).

Elderly patients are sensitive to the side-effects of lithium and at greater risk of neurotoxicity. The elderly may experience lithium toxicity when plasma levels are within the therapeutic range. Up to 50% of elderly patients will experience side-effects with lithium (Flint and Rifat 1994). Tables 4.6 and 4.7 list the common side-effects of lithium and signs of toxicity. The elderly may respond to lower plasma concentrations of lithium than younger patients, although Flint (1995) suggests levels of greater than 0.5 mmol/L are necessary. In a review of lithium use in the elderly, Foster (1992) suggested an ideal range of 0.4–0.7 mmol/L. Once-daily dosing minimizes side-effects.

Initial reports of lithium augmentation suggested that a response occurred within a few days, but 3–4 weeks is considered a minimum trial. It is important to monitor elderly patients on lithium closely and to adhere to guidelines on monitoring. The British National Formulary (1999) advises examining lithium levels every 3 months if dose and physical health are stable. After

Table 4.6. Common non-toxic side-effects of lithium in older people (Foster 1992).

Side-effect	Approximate range of patients experiencing side-effect (%)
Polydipsia	50–74
Polyuria	25–58
Tremor	33–58
Dry mouth	53
Nausea	33

Table 4.7. Symptoms and signs of lithium toxicity.

Coarse tremor
Ataxia/falls
Blurred vision
Weakness
Drowsiness
Increasing gastrointestinal disturbance
Slurred speech
Nystagmus

Signs of neurotoxicity usually develop when plasma levels are greater than 1.5 mmol/L but may occur at lithium levels within the therapeutic range in the elderly, especially during periods of physical illness.

starting lithium or any change in dose, plasma concentrations should be checked at 4–7 days, and then weekly until stable. Closer monitoring may be warranted for some elderly patients, particularly those with a history of heart disease or renal impairment. Important in reducing the risk of toxicity is giving patients and carers clear and preferably written information about lithium and ensuring that this information is understood.

Patients at particular risk of lithium toxicity are those taking thiazide diuretics (25% reduction in lithium excretion) or non-steroidal anti-inflammatory drugs. Toxicity can occur if the risks of drug–lithium interactions are not fully recognized and drugs are started which interact with lithium without checking lithium levels. Commonly prescribed drugs in the elderly which may lead to an increase in lithium concentration are angiotensin-converting enzyme inhibitors, thiazide diuretics and NSAIDs. Of the NSAIDs, Sulindac may be the safest (Bazire 1998). Aspirin is probably safe to use with lithium as there was little effect on lithium concentrations in one study. Patients should be warned not to buy ibuprofen over the counter without discussing this with their GP.

There is little evidence to guide clinicians on how long lithium augmentation should be continued once a response has been achieved. Risks of long-term lithium maintenance have to be weighed against the risks of recurrence of a mood disorder for each patient. Maintenance treatment with lithium is associated with hypothyroidism so regular monitoring of thyroid function is necessary. In one survey 25% of patients on maintenance lithium were also taking thyroxine (Head and Denning 1998). Urea and electrolytes with serum creatinine should also be monitored. Therapeutic levels of lithium are not thought to lead to renal impairment but episodes of toxicity may cause renal damage. Renal impairment due to other causes significantly increases the risk of toxicity (Case History 4.4).

The addition of tri-iodothyronine (T_3) to antidepressant medication at doses of 25–50 µg per day is a strategy that has been used in younger patients with treatment-resistant depression. A meta-analysis of eight controlled studies, mainly involving younger patients, showed that T_3 augmentation

Case History 4.4

An 80-year-old man was admitted urgently to a psychiatric ward. He had become increasingly depressed and withdrawn over 3 months despite treatment with fluoxetine 20 mg daily. On the day of admission he had expressed thoughts of suicide. He had been well in the past apart from hypertension for which he was prescribed bendrofluazide.

The fluoxetine was stopped and he was commenced on lofepramine and the dose increased to 210 mg daily. There was no improvement after 4 weeks and he agreed to ECT. He was given a total of 12 treatments without effect. Lithium augmentation was considered and his bendrofluazide was stopped and blood pressure monitored. Within 2 weeks of commencing lithium mood responded and after a month his mood returned to normal. A year later he remained well on lithium carbonate 400 mg daily.

produced twice as many responses as controls (Aronson *et al.* 1996). There have been no controlled studies of T_3 augmentation in elderly patients (Flint 1995) and so routine use in the elderly cannot be justified, although it may be of benefit in individual cases. The British National Formulary (1999) advises caution in using T_3 augmentation in the elderly, especially those with cardio-vascular disease. Small doses of T_3 should be used with regular monitoring of thyroid function, aiming to double free thyroid hormone levels.

Open studies and case series have reported responses in elderly patients to augmentation with carbamazepine and sodium valproate in treatment-resistant depression (Flint 1995). The use of carbamazepine and sodium valproate as mood stabilizers in bipolar affective disorder is well established, but as yet there is no evidence of their efficacy from randomized controlled studies in treatment-resistant depression in the elderly (Baldwin 1999). They should therefore be used with caution in the elderly. Carbamazepine has lim-iting side-effects in the elderly, including drowsiness, nausea and ataxia and regular blood tests are necessary as there is a risk of blood dyscrasias (British National Formulary 1999). Sodium valproate seems to be better tolerated in the elderly (Flint 1995).

Other augmentation strategies that have been used in younger patients are listed in Table 4.8. Apart from the use of antipsychotic medication in psychotic depression (Flint and Rifat 1998), evidence from randomized controlled trials of their efficacy in the elderly is lacking. They may be considered in some patients where other strategies have failed.

Key points

- Although important, the pharmacological treatment of depression in older people should form part of an overall management plan which considers and addresses psychosocial factors and non-pharmacological treatments.
- Older people are more sensitive to the side-effects of medication because of pharmacodynamic and pharmacokinetic changes with age. Medication should be started at low dose and increased gradually.
- Evidence from randomized controlled trials suggests that antidepressants are of equal efficacy as first-line pharmacotherapy in the treatment of non-psychotic depression. Choice of antidepressant is usually governed by the avoidance of side-effects and drug interactions.
- Response to antidepressants is slower or delayed in the elderly. However, if there is no response to an initial antidepressant after 4 weeks a change to a different class of antidepressant should be considered. If there is a partial response at 4 weeks the antidepressant can be continued with regular mon-itoring of the mental state. If subsequent response is slow or incomplete ECT or augmentation should be considered.
- If there is no response to pharmacotherapy the diagnosis should be reviewed. Poor compliance with medication and adverse psychosocial fac-tors should be addressed before making changes to pharmacotherapy.
- The risk of recurrence is high following an episode of depression in the

Table 4.8. Alternative augmentation strategies in treatment-resistant depression.

Strategy	Rationale	Evidence of efficacy	Side-effects and cautions
Tryptophan	Precursor to serotonin	Used in combination with TCAs and lithium. Evidence of use in elderly is lacking.	Eosinophilia–myalgia syndrome reported. Eosinophil count monitoring necessary.
Antidepressant combinations	Increase in antidepressant serum levels	One study showed marginal benefit only (O'Brien et al. 1993). Case reports of improvement in elderly with refractory depression.	Combinations are potentially hazardous. Usual combination of SSRI with low dose TCA. Risk of serotonin syndrome or delirium in the elderly.
Antipsychotics	Sedative Anxiolytic	Augmentation strategy of choice if depression complicated by psychotic symptoms. (Baldwin 1988).	Extra-pyramidal side-effects. TCA levels increased by antipsychotics.
Pindolol	Blocks pre-synaptic inhibitory 5-HT receptors. Increases 5-HT in synaptic cleft when combined with serotinergic antidepressants	Out of six controlled studies, only three showed any benefit (McAskill et al. 1998). No studies of efficacy in the elderly.	Controlled studies report few side-effects or adverse events.

elderly. To reduce this high risk of recurrence pharmacotherapy should be continued for at least 1 year after recovery and preferably 2 years. Longer continuation treatment should be considered for those older patients with a history of recurrent depression.

References

Alexopoulos, G.S., Meyers, B.S., Young, R.C., Campbell, S., Silbersweig, D. and Charlson, M. (1997) 'Vascular depression' hypothesis. *Archives of General Psychiatry*, **54**, 915–922.

Anderson, I.M. and Tomenson, B.M. (1995) Treatment discontinuation with selective serotonin reuptake inhibitors compared with tricyclic antidepressants: a meta-analysis. *British Medical Journal*, **310**, 1433–1438.

Aronson, R., Offman, H.J., Joffe, R.T. and Naylor, C.D. (1996) Triiodothyronine augmentation in the treatment of refractory depression: a meta-analysis. *Archives of General Psychiatry*, **53**, 842–848.

Baldwin, R.C. (1999) Delusional and non-delusional depression in late life: evidence of distinct subtypes. *British Journal of Psychiatry*, **152**, 39–44.

Baldwin, R. and Burns, A. (1999) Pharmacological treatments. In *Seminars in Old Age Psychiatry*, edited by R. Butler and B. Pitt, pp. 247–264. Gaskell, London.

Bazire, S. (1998) *Psychotropic Drug Directory*. Quay Books, Salisbury, Wilts.

Bertilsson, L. and Dahl, M. L. (1996) Polymorphic drug oxidation: relevance to treatment of psychiatric disorders. *CNS Drugs*, **3**, 200–223.

Bridges, P. K., Hodgkiss, A.D. and Malizia, A.L. (1995) Practical management of treatment-resistant affective disorders. *British Journal of Hospital Medicine*, **54**, 501–506.

British National Formulary 37 (1999) British Medical Association.

Buckley, N.A., Dawson, A.H., Whyte, I.M. and Henry, D.A. (1994) Greater toxicity in overdose of dothiepin than other tricyclic antidepressants. *The Lancet*, **343**, 159–162.

Curran, S. and Freeman, C.P. (1995) ECT and drugs. In *The ECT Handbook*, edited by C.P. Freeman, pp. 49–57. The Royal College of Psychiatrists, London.

Drugs and Therapeutics Bulletin (1999) Withdrawing patients from antidepressants. *Drugs and Therapeutics Bulletin*, **37**, 49–52.

Edwards, J.G. (1995) Suicide and antidepressants. Editorial. *British Medical Journal*, **310**, 205–206.

Flint, A.J. (1992) The optimum duration of antidepressant treatment in the elderly. *International Journal of Geriatric Psychiatry*, **7**, 617–619.

Flint, A.J. (1995) Augmentation strategies in geriatric depression. *International Journal of Geriatric Psychiatry*, **10**, 137–146.

Flint, A.J. and Rifat, S.L. (1994) A prospective study of lithium augmentation in antidepressant-resistant geriatric depression. *Journal of Clinical Psychopharmacology*, **14**, 353–356.

Flint, A.J. and Rifat, S.L. (1998) The treatment of psychotic depression in later life: a comparison of pharmacotherapy and ECT. *International Journal of Geriatric Psychiatry*, **13**, 23–28.

Foster, J.R. (1992) Use of lithium in elderly psychiatric patients: a review of the literature. *Lithium*, **3**, 77–93.

Frank, E., Kupfer, D.J., Perel, J.M., Cornes, C., Jarrett, D.B., Mallinger, A.G. *et al.*

(1990) Three year outcomes for maintenance therapies in recurrent depression. *Archives of General Psychiatry*, **47**, 1093–1099.

Georgetas, A. and McCue, R. (1989) The additional benefit of extending an antidepressant trial past seven weeks in the depressed elderly. *International Journal of Geriatric Psychiatry*, **4**, 191–195.

Head, L. and Denning, T. (1998) Lithium in the over-65s: who is taking it and who is monitoring it? *International Journal of Geriatric Psychiatry*, **13**, 164–171.

Hotopf, M., Hardy, R. and Lewis, G. (1997) Discontinuation rates of SSRIs and tricyclic antidepressants: a meta-analysis and investigation of heterogeneity. *British Journal of Psychiatry*, **170**, 120–127.

Lader, M. (1994) Neuropharmacology and pharmacokinetics of psychotropic drugs in old age. In *Principles and Practice of Geriatric Psychiatry*, edited by J. Copeland, M. Abou-Saleh and D. Blazer, pp. 79–82. John Wiley, Chichester.

Livingston, G.L. and Livingston, M.L. (1999) New antidepressants for old people? Editorial. *British Medical Journal*, **318**, 1640–1641.

McAskill, R., Mir, S. and Taylor, D. (1998) Pindolol augmentation of antidepressant therapy. *British Journal of Psychiatry*, **173**, 203–208.

O'Brien, S., McKeown, P. and O'Ryan, M. (1993) The efficacy and tolerability of combined antidepressant treatment in different depressive subgroups. *British Journal of Psychiatry*, **162**, 363–368.

Old Age Depression Interest Group (OADIG) (1993) How long should the elderly take antidepressants? A double blind placebo controlled study continuation/prophylaxis therapy with dothiepin. *British Journal of Psychiatry*, **162**, 175–182.

Prien, R.F. and Kupfer, D.J. (1986) Continuation drug therapy for major depressive episodes: how long should it be maintained? *American Journal of Psychiatry*, **143**, 18–23.

Quitkin, F.M., Robkin, J.G., Ross, D. and McGrath, P. J. (1984) Duration of antidepressant drug treatment. *Archives of General Psychiatry*, **41**, 238–245.

Roose, S.P. , Glassman, A.H., Attia, E. and Woodring, S. (1994) Comparative efficacy of selective serotonin reuptake inhibitors and tricyclics in the treatment of melancholia. *American Journal of Psychiatry*, **151**, 1735–1739.

Roth, M., Mountjoy, C.Q., Amrein, R. and the International Collaborative Study Group (1996) Moclobemide in elderly patients with cognitive decline and depression. *British Journal of Psychiatry*, **168**, 149–157.

Song, F., Freemantle, N., Sheldon, T.A., House, A., Watson, P. , Long, A. *et al.* (1993) Selective serotonin reuptake inhibitors: meta-analysis of efficacy and acceptability. *British Medical Journal*, **306**, 683–687.

Spigset, O. and Martensson, B. (1999) Drug treatment of depression. *British Medical Journal*, **318**, 1188–1191.

Spiker, D.G., Weiss, J.C., Dealy, R.S., Griffin, S.J., Hanin, I., Neil, J.F. *et al.* (1985) The pharmacological treatment of delusional depression. *American Journal of Psychiatry*, **142**, 430–436.

Taylor, D., McConnell, D., McConnell, H. and Abel, K. (1999) *The Bethlem and Maudsley NHS Trust Prescribing Guidelines*. Martin Dunitz, London.

Wattis, J., Bentham, P. and Bestley, J. (1994) Choice of antidepressants by psychiatrists working with old people. *Psychiatric Bulletin*, **18**, 148–151.

ECT in the treatment of depression in older people

Susan Benbow

Introduction

Electroconvulsive therapy (ECT) has been used in psychiatry for over 50 years, but, despite a wealth of papers on the subject, it still arouses controversy (Fink 1991). Brandt and Ugarriza (1996) examined the myths about ECT and pointed out that it carries considerable social stigma, so that many people keep their experience of it secret. They concluded that there is a need for public education to tackle deficits in knowledge and dispel myths.

When Pippard and Ellam (1981) carried out a national survey of ECT usage in Great Britain they found that 37% of courses were given to people aged over 60 years of age. In 1985 alone 137 940 ECT treatments were administered in England, with a steady but slowing decline to a reported total of 105 466 treatments in 1990–1991 (Department of Health 1992). The national average rate at that time was 220 treatments per 100 000 population. From January 1999 to March 1999 the Department of Health (1999) surveyed the use of ECT in England and reported on 16 500 treatments administered to 2800 individuals. Forty-four per cent of the women treated were over 65 years of age and 33% of the men. These figures translate to an estimated 65 930 treatments per full year and show that those over 65 years of age remain major users of ECT services. In 1995 the mental health charity MIND published a report on older women and ECT (Cobb 1995) and campaigned for a scaling down of its use, arguing that older women are over-represented amongst the population of people treated with ECT. There are, however, a number of possible reasons why older people might be more likely to require ECT. In the past it has been assumed that the increased use of ECT in older people might relate to their increased sensitivity to the side-effects of older antidepressants, but Olfson *et al.* (1998) argue that this can no longer be the case with the advent of newer antidepressant drugs. It may relate to difference in patients' attitudes towards, or acceptance of, the treatment, or 'entrenched practice patterns'. They also note that there is some data suggesting that older depressed adults may preferentially respond to ECT rather than antidepressant drugs.

Case History 5.1a

Mrs Ethel King, widow, born 1909, was first referred by her GP to the old age psychiatry service in January 1991 for home assessment. She had an agitated depressive illness with classical biological symptoms of depression and suicidal ideas. She had written what appeared to be a suicide note to her daughter. There was no previous history of psychiatric illness. Her husband had died 2 years earlier and she had been first observed by the family to be depressed about 6 months previously. The week before referral her baby grandson had died. She agreed to admission to a psychiatric ward for treatment and was already on a tricyclic antidepressant initiated by the general practitioner. Within a few hours of admission she collapsed and was transferred to a medical ward, where she was diagnosed as having a chest infection, with atrial fibrillation and heart failure. Following medical treatment she was transferred back to the psychiatric ward. The tricyclic was continued throughout this illness and the dose gradually increased. She improved steadily and made a full recovery. After a series of successful home visits she was discharged home to attend a local day centre for 2 days each week.

Regular follow up was carried out by a community psychiatric nurse and in the community clinic and she remained well on antidepressants until June 1993 when, on a routine visit, she was noted to have low mood with diurnal variation. She dated the onset of symptoms to the recent anniversary of her husband's death. The frequency of visits was increased and she complied with antidepressant drug treatment, but her mood continued to deteriorate. She was re-admitted in August 1993. She was drowsy and the tricyclic antidepressant was changed, but she showed no response to a therapeutic dose and agreed to a course of ECT. She made an excellent recovery with nine bilateral ECT and was discharged home on a different class of antidepressant, a selective serotonin re-uptake inhibitor

(Whilst this case describes a person under my care, the name and some of the details have been changed to prevent identification.)

Indications for ECT

Most older people treated with ECT have a severe depressive illness, particularly depressive illness with psychotic symptoms. This was regarded as the main indication in a survey of the views of old age psychiatrists (Benbow 1991). Other diagnostic groupings where ECT was rated as 'often' or 'sometimes' useful by over 50% of respondents were schizoaffective disorder and depressive illness with dementia. The same study investigated the circumstances in which ECT might be the treatment of choice in old age psychiatry and over 50% of respondents supported its use in the following situations:

- depressive illness which has failed to respond to antidepressant drugs;
- depressive illness where previous episodes responded to ECT but not to antidepressant drugs;
- depressive illness with psychotic symptoms;
- depressive illness with severe agitation;
- depressive illness with high suicidal risk; and
- depressive stupor.

When Mrs King received her first course of ECT (Case History 5.1a) she had relapsed on one antidepressant drug and had failed to respond to therapeutic doses of a second. She had marked biological symptoms of depression and in the past the symptoms associated with the classical concept of 'endogenous depression' have been regarded as predictors of a good response to treatment (Benbow 1989).

Case History 5.1b

Follow-up visits found Mrs King to be well, living independently and with no depressive symptoms. But in January 1997 she suddenly presented with a relapse of agitated depressive illness and was admitted for the third time. In view of the history of good response to ECT and relapse on antidepressant drug treatment she was offered, and accepted, a course of ECT. She received 10 bilateral ECT treatments, made a good recovery and was discharged home after a graded discharge programme on a selective serotonin re-uptake inhibitor and lithium carbonate. At follow-up review in the community there were no depressive symptoms.

Technical aspects of ECT practice

Bilateral electrode placement is preferable for people whose concurrent medical conditions make it advisable to minimize the number of general anaesthetics. For this reason Mrs King was treated with bilateral ECT (Case History 5.1b). Unilateral electrode placement is indicated for people with pre-existing cognitive impairment, in order to minimize cognitive side-effects during treatment (Benbow 1995).

The ECT Handbook (Freeman 1995) does not recommend the use of stimulus dosing but gives guidelines on how to design a stimulus dosing policy, and gives examples of protocols to use with different ECT machines. Stimulus dosing refers to adjusting the dose of electricity used for ECT to the individual being treated in order that it exceeds the individual's seizure threshold by an amount which should be effective without incurring excessive adverse cognitive side-effects. The dosing strategy in an ECT clinic needs to take into account differences between individual patients and changes within an individual across a course of treatment. This may involve using tables, which take account of age and gender, to pre-determine the initial electrical dose, or using a protocol to titrate a gradually increasing dose of electricity until a dose is found that elicits a seizure (Lock 1995). Treatment dose will be determined by a protocol in relation to the seizure threshold (Table 5.1). One of these protocols was in use in the ECT clinic where Mrs King had her second course of ECT and Table 5.1 shows how the dose was increased over the first two sessions in order to determine an approximation of seizure threshold (in this case 151 mC).

The treatment dose was administered subsequently at a level between 50 and 100% above seizure threshold. Higher seizure thresholds are related to increasing age, and to male gender. Various drug treatments can also raise seizure threshold and/or shorten seizure duration. These may be important considerations in deciding on drug treatments during ECT for older adults who tend to have higher seizure thresholds in any case, especially older men. Table 5.2 sets out factors which influence seizure threshold or duration.

ECT itself is a powerful anti-convulsant and Table 5.1 shows how Mrs King's treatment dose was increased after her sixth treatment because of shortening of the cerebral seizure activity (as recorded on EEG monitoring), which is presumed to be secondary to increasing seizure threshold as treatment proceeded.

Table 5.1. Details of Mrs King's second course of ECT (bilateral).

Treatment number	Stimulus (mC)	EEG end-point (s)	Motor activity (s)	Comments
1	(1) 76	(1) no CSA*	(1) 0	Increasing stimulus as per the dosing protocol to determine seizure threshold
	(2) 101	(2) NO CSA	(2) 0	
	(3) 353	(3) 72	(3) 58	
2	151	51	30	Seizure threshold
3	252	60	52	Treatment dose
4	252	51	42	–
5	252	48	39	–
6	252	40	27	Shortening of seizure over treatments 3 to 6–dose increased next treatment
7	353	62	39	
8	353	66	31	
9	353	85	37	
10	353	83	44	

*CSA, cerebral seizure activity.

Table 5.2. Factors influencing seizure threshold and/or duration.

Factor	Details
Gender	ST* higher in men
Electrode placement	ST in bilateral placement higher than unilateral
Age	ST increases with age
Anaesthetic drugs	Raise threshold and/or shorten duration
Psychotropic drugs	Raise threshold and/or shorten duration, e.g. Benzodiazepines, L-tryptophan
Other drugs	(1) Some lower threshold and/or lengthen duration, e.g. caffeine, theophylline, reserpine. Caffeine is sometimes used pre-ECT in people with high seizure threshold. (2) Some raise threshold and/or shorten duration, e.g. anticoagulants, beta-blockers.
ECT	ECT itself increases ST
Hyperventilation/ hyperoxygenation	Can be used to lengthen seizure duration during treatment in people having short seizures.

*ST = seizure threshold.

Case History 5.1c: rapid post-operative relapse

At the end of August 1997 Mrs King fell at home and fractured her femur. Pre-operatively her mood was noted to be good but immediately post-operatively a marked change was observed. She appeared low, was uncommunicative, and refused food, drink and medication. On the surgical ward nurses resorted to syringing fluids into her mouth. She was assessed by a physician who could find no physical reason for the deterioration. Her psychoactive drugs had been discontinued on admission and she was referred for psychiatric assessment 10 days post-operation. Assessment supported a diagnosis of severe depressive illness and, after due consultation, Section 3 of the Mental Health Act was implemented since, because she was mute, she could not consent to ECT and was only drinking and eating with much nursing effort. A Second Opinion Appointed Doctor supported the plan to treat her with a course of up to 12 ECT treatments and treatment was started without delay.

Consent to ECT

Martin and Bean (1992) examined the issues associated with competence to consent from a North American perspective, pointing out that there are no pass/fail criteria for competence and that capacity is an elusive concept. Consent is a continuous dynamic process and this is fundamentally true of consent to ECT. People who have consented may withdraw their consent at any time and, because depressive illnesses in late life may affect cognition, as indeed may ECT, it will be necessary to provide repeated explanations as people proceed with their treatment.

Older adults who are being advised to consent to ECT will need to be provided with information about the treatment (nature, purposes, effects and side-effects), about why it is being suggested and what the alternatives are.

They will need time to think it over, to discuss the decision with staff and relatives, and to ask questions. It is good practice to use written information about treatment in addition to verbal explanation. (The CRAG working group on Mental Illness (1997) produced a good practice statement which includes a Patient Information Leaflet about ECT and a sheet for people receiving ECT as outpatients.)

In some circumstances people will be unable to consent to ECT. This was clearly the case with Mrs King who was mute and unable to co-operate post-operatively. The relevant Mental Health Act procedures will need to be used in these circumstances. If an informal but capable patient refuses consent to ECT, alternative treatments will need to be considered unless there are grounds for invoking the Mental Health Act. A procedure for making a decision on behalf of those unable to consent is vitally important since severe depression may affect capacity. A person who believes that everything is hopeless and that they would be better off dead may be unable to conceive of these ideas arising from a treatable illness. The right to treatment despite being unable to consent is a fundamental human right and society has a responsibility on behalf of its most vulnerable members to allow them the possibility of recovery.

Case History 5.1d: a third course of ECT

The third course of treatment was interrupted, first by an episode of paroxysmal atrial fibrillation, and later when she became dehydrated in response to over-diuresis. After 12 ECT treatments she was bright, communicative, interactive and mobilizing independently, but with persistent low mood in the mornings. She consented to a further six ECT treatments (i.e. a total of 18) and gradually recovered. During the course of treatments 13 to 18 she had a bout of confusion secondary to a urinary tract infection: this was treated with a course of antibiotics, and she was restarted on lithium treatment.

Safety of ECT

Adverse effects of ECT

ECT is a low-risk procedure with a mortality similar to anaesthesia for minor surgical procedures: approximately 2 deaths per 100 000 treatments. After treatment people may suffer from:

- headaches;
- muscular aches;
- drowsiness;
- weakness;
- nausea; and
- anorexia.

These are usually only mild and respond to symptomatic treatments. Other side-effects include:

- cognitive side-effects;
- acute confusion; and
- adverse psychological reactions.

Cognitive side-effects are the main concern in older people, and have been extensively studied. ECT can affect memory for events which occurred before ECT (retrograde amnesia) and events which take place after ECT (anterograde amnesia). The ability to learn new information and non-memory cognitive functions (including intelligence, judgement, abstraction, etc.) are not affected. Severe depressive illness, particularly in older adults, can affect memory and tests of memory carried out before and after ECT may show improvement, presumably because the memory deficits associated with depression have improved in response to treatment. Objective memory impairment (that is impairment which can be demonstrated on objective tests) occurring during a course of ECT is reversible, and no objective deficits have been demonstrated in the small proportion of people who complain of persisting memory difficulty after treatment, Some of these may have chronic depressive symptoms. Fink (1999) argues that depressive illness and psychotropic drugs affect memory, but that when ECT is used detrimental effects are blamed solely on the ECT which then bears 'the full burden of the public's fear of every psychiatric treatment's cognitive effects'.

Acute confusional states may develop between treatments, particularly in people taking concurrent psychotropic drugs, or those with pre-existing cognitive impairment or neurological conditions. If this occurs, modifications to treatment technique may lessen the confusion. Rarely a person will develop post-ictal delirium which can manifest as restlessness, aggression or agitation in the early stages of recovery. This will respond to treatment with benzodiazepines.

Adverse psychological reactions to ECT may involve the person developing an intense fear of treatment. Support and information is critical in preventing and managing this side-effect of treatment.

Concurrent physical illness

There are no absolute contraindications to ECT (Fink 1999). People with a wide range of physical illnesses have been successfully treated with ECT. For any individual the potential risks and benefits need to be assessed before making a decision regarding whether or not to go ahead with treatment, and medical treatment may need to be optimized first. Careful explanation will help the patient and their relatives to understand treatment options and allow an informed decision. Medical problems which cause particular difficulty include *cardiovascular disease* and *neurological conditions*.

CARDIOVASCULAR DISEASE

People with cardiovascular disease are at increased risk of cardiac complications during ECT. Complications during ECT increase with the age of recipients and Burke *et al.* (1987) reported increased complications in people on a greater total number of medications and in those on a greater number of cardiovascular medications. Zielinski *et al.* (1998) found that most cardiovascular complications were transient and did not prevent successful completion of the treatment course, concluding that ECT can be used relatively safely for people with severe cardiac disease.

Blood pressure and heart rate fall during the passage of the electrical stimulus and then rise rapidly. Cerebral blood flow and cerebrovascular permeability increase, with a sudden short-lived increase in intra-cranial pressure. A sinus bradycardia results initially from vagal stimulation, sometimes with periods of electrical silence (asystole), but is rapidly replaced by a marked tachycardia mediated by sympathetic neurones. Tachycardia can cause ischaemia by decreasing myocardial oxygen supply and increasing oxygen consumption. Sub-convulsive stimuli produce longer periods of bradycardia, which may be a concern when people with known heart disease are treated using a protocol involving dose titration to determine seizure threshold (Abrams 1991, Dolinski and Zvara 1997). Beta blockers are another risk factor for longer periods of asystole during ECT (McCall 1996).

Abrams (1997a) states that the 'detection and management of significant cardiovascular disease before administering ECT . . . is . . . the most important factor in reducing . . . cardiovascular morbidity and mortality'. He reviews its use in conjunction with cardiac pacemakers, aortic aneurysms, previous cardiac surgery, myocardial infarction and intra-cardiac thrombi, and the use of agents to reduce blood pressure or reduce heart rate and prevent arrhythmias.

NEUROLOGICAL CONDITIONS

People who have space occupying lesions of the brain are at high risk of neurological deterioration if treated with ECT, although it has been used safely for people with small slow-growing tumours unassociated with raised intra-cranial pressure. The risk is thought to be associated with aggravation of already raised intra-cranial pressure (Abrams 1997a).

ECT has been used successfully in people with a wide range of neurological conditions including cerebral vascular malformations, following stroke, following craniotomy, in the presence of concurrent dementia, learning disability, lupus cerebritis or epilepsy. Prior to ECT the underlying disorder is fully assessed and treated and the risks explained to the patient. In liaison with the anaesthetist treatment technique may be modified to minimize the risks involved (Benbow 1995).

OTHER MEDICAL CONDITIONS

Use of muscle relaxant drugs has virtually eliminated the risk of fracture during ECT. Intra-occular pressure rises transiently during ECT, but this is only a concern in people with advanced glaucoma, for whom ophthalmological advice should be sought (Abrams 1997a).

CLINICAL RELEVANCE TO THIS PATIENT

Mrs King was known to have ischaemic heart disease before she started this course of ECT and was therefore at increased risk of cardiac complications. She developed an arrhythmia (paroxysmal atrial fibrillation) immediately after her third treatment, but was able to continue the course. She also became dehydrated and had a urinary tract infection. This clustering of physical problems during a course of treatment is probably not uncommon in old age psychiatry and illustrates both the complexity of treating an older adult with multiple problems and the fact that despite the difficulties treatment can still lead to recovery.

Case History 5.1e: another rapid release

Within 3 weeks of the latest ECT, Mrs King was noted by nursing staff to be increasingly lethargic, increasingly reluctant to eat and drink, less communicative, avoiding eye contact, and spontaneously saying that she felt fed up and wished she were dead. A further urinary tract infection was diagnosed and in view of the bouts of confusion a CT brain scan was carried out. It was reported to show 'diffuse cerebrovascular disease' with areas of focal infarction. Mrs King's mood continued to deteriorate and, after discussion with the family and Mrs King herself, a further course of unilateral ECT was commenced in early February 1998.

ECT and dementia

ECT has been rated as appropriate 'often' or 'sometimes' in the treatment of depressive illness with a concurrent dementia (Benbow 1991). Some psychiatrists are nevertheless cautious about using ECT when a person has an established diagnosis of dementia and people may have to seek actively for a clinic prepared to treat them, even though they have a clear history of ECT responsive recurrent depressive illnesses. In a previous local audit (Benbow 1992) one-quarter of patients treated consecutively under the care of one old age psychiatrist had a concurrent dementing illness. People with co-existing dementia were found to be more likely to be treated under the Mental Health Act (presumably because of difficulties in ensuring informed consent) and were more likely to develop confusion lasting more than 48 hours during their course of treatment. They were more likely to be partial responders to treatment, rather than make a complete recovery, but this may reflect the difficulty of assessing improvement in people with an underlying dementia. They were just as likely as people without dementia to be discharged home.

Unilateral ECT may be advisable in this group in order to minimize cognitive side-effects during treatment and careful ongoing monitoring of cognitive function during treatment is wise, with close attention to any factors which might decrease the severity of any adverse effect on cognition. This would include minimizing the dose of anaesthetic, avoiding concurrent drug treatments which might exacerbate confusion, and using a dosing schedule to tailor the dose to the individual. After Mrs King had been found to have cerebrovascular disease, she was treated with unilateral ECT.

Case History 5.1f: unilateral treatment

After only three treatments Mrs King was starting to improve again, being more 'with it' and brighter in mood. Her maintenance drug treatment was changed to a tricyclic antidepressant and lithium but she developed difficulties in passing urine and the tricyclic was changed. Treatment frequency was decreased from twice to once weekly as she recovered, then to once every 10 days and eventually once every 2 weeks. Meanwhile she went on a series of home visits which culminated in Mrs King accepting that she could no longer live alone and would like to move into a residential home near her daughter. After 18 ECT she was discharged to a Rest Home in June 1998, euthymic, and agreeing to continue with maintenance ECT, then at a frequency of once every 2 weeks. She was also taking lithium and a tricyclic antidepressant.

Close follow-up continued after discharge. Mrs King's mood remained good and the ECT interval was lengthened to three-weekly. In December 1998 she developed an eye infection, her maintenance treatment was cancelled and she became acutely depressed, culminating in readmission late that month. She was treated on admission for a chest infection and then consented to restart ECT, initially unilateral ECT twice weekly but changing to bilateral ECT in view of poor initial response. Subsequently the interval between treatments was gradually lengthened. At discharge in March 1999 she was having one bilateral treatment every 10–14 days and remained on lithium and an antidepressant. After discharge maintenance treatment continued and the interval between treatments 6 months later was 2 weeks.

Maintenance ECT

Maintenance ECT (M-ECT) is an empirically developed treatment. Kendell (1981) stated that there is only rarely need for M-ECT, but a later national survey by Pippard and Ellam (1981) reported that 22% of their respondents used M-ECT. Kramer (1987) surveyed ECT practitioner members of the International Psychiatric Association for the Advancement of Electrotherapy, a majority of whom practised in the USA, and found that 59% indicated that they used some form of M-ECT with a median of three individuals over the previous 3 years.

In terms of definition, treatments intended to prevent relapse (continuation treatments) can be distinguished (at least in theory) from treatments to prevent recurrent episodes of illness. Thus continuation ECT (C-ECT) can be distinguished from maintenance ECT (M-ECT), although in practice it might be debatable how helpful this distinction is, since continuation often blurs into maintenance treatment; the suggested cut-off of 6 months when C-ECT transforms into M-ECT is arbitrary.

The American Psychiatric Association Recommendations (1990) cover both continuation and maintenance treatment. Continuation therapy is defined as beginning when therapeutic intent shifts from active treatment to prevention of relapse, and the recommendations state that it should be continued for at least 6 months. Maintenance therapy is defined as treatment continuing for longer than 6 months following completion of the most recent ECT course and aims to prevent recurrence of new episodes of the index disorder. Criteria for patient selection are set out. For C-ECT these are three-fold: history of recurrent episodes responsive to ECT, and either failure of pharmacotherapy to prevent relapse, or patient preference, and agreement from the patient to C-ECT. M-ECT is regarded as indicated when a need for maintenance treatment exists in people who are already receiving C-ECT, and the American Psychiatric Association (APA) states that the frequency of treatment should be the minimum compatible with sustained remission, generally one treatment every 1–3 months, with reassessment every 3 months.

These recommendations are similar to those in the Royal College of Psychiatrists ECT Handbook (Scott 1995). The three criteria for considering C-ECT listed by Scott are similar to those of the APA: an ECT-responsive index illness; early relapse despite continuation drug treatment (or inability to tolerate continuation drug treatment); patient's attitude and circumstances conducive to safe administration. Scott notes that C-ECT may be appropriate at any age, although many reports concern older people. He comments on the need to titrate treatment frequency according to individual need, to assess memory regularly throughout treatment and to minimize concomitant drug treatment. Monroe (1991) distinguished two distinct populations which might benefit from M-ECT (those intolerant of pharmacotherapy and those with relapsing/psychotic depression) and two types of treatment schedules, tapered schedules (where the interval between treatments extends as the treatment continues) and indefinite fixed dose schedules.

Much of the literature concerning M-ECT and C-ECT is largely historical and quite unlike present day practice. Stevenson and Geoghegan (1951) described treatment schedules which started with monthly treatment for 5 years, then decreased to 2–monthly, then 3–monthly and finally 6–monthly. A more recent schedule for continuation treatment described by Clarke *et al.* (1989) starts with weekly ECT for 1 month, biweekly ECT for a second month and thereafter monthly ECT.

Older age groups tend to predominate in studies of M-ECT (Duncan *et al.* (1990) described a 90–year-old treated with M-ECT over 16 months), but many studies have been based on small sample sizes.

Attempts have been made to study efficacy by comparing rates of psychiatric hospital admission before and after starting M-ECT. Schwarz *et al.* (1995) compared 21 patients with unipolar or bipolar depressive illnesses who received M-ECT with two other groups, one of whom received ECT but did not progress to maintenance treatment and the other of whom received pharmacotherapy alone. The average course of M-ECT was eight treatments administered over 6 months. M-ECT was found to be used in people with a course of multiple hospital admissions and established failure to respond to other therapies: on average they had been exposed to 10 different psychotropic medications prior to M-ECT and this included an average five trials of tricyclic antidepressants. Vanelle *et al.* (1994) studied 22 people suffering from intractable recurrent unipolar or bipolar mood disorders who enrolled in an M-ECT programme for more than 18 months. They were treated approximately monthly and 11 continued with treatment for over 2 years. Prior to M-ECT the group spent 44% of the year in hospital, averaging three episodes per year, but afterwards they had only one relapse every 16 months and spent 7% of the year in hospital. These differences were found to be highly significant. Illnesses with psychotic symptoms appeared to respond best and organic brain syndromes were not regarded as a contraindication to maintenance treatment.

Other issues of relevance to the use of M-ECT in later life include the potential physical risk of repeated anaesthetics, the potential risk of cognitive impairment and the role of pharmacotherapy.

Mrs King had relapsed on two separate antidepressants and on combination treatment (with lithium) before she received M-ECT. One of the practical problems in treating her has been how to determine the frequency of treatment. This has been done by empirical titration, by monitoring her response and the emergence of any depressive symptoms, particularly diurnal mood variation, as her relapses have been heralded by low mood and weepiness in the early morning. Very few people receive M-ECT so the experience of any individual psychiatrist will be limited. In a study of psychiatrists in Northwest England, 25% (30) of respondents stated that they used M-ECT and 67% (82) that they would be prepared to consider using M-ECT. Forty-nine per cent of the respondents stated that they had not prescribed maintenance treatment within the past 10 years. Recurrent depressive illness was the most common diagnosis amongst people prescribed M-ECT. Dementia was not generally regarded as a contraindication to the use of M-ECT, nor was advanced age. Most respondents prescribed M-ECT on a variable regime for up to 12 months, using bilateral electrode placement with continuation of prophylactic mood-stabilizing drugs.

In summary, throughout Mrs King's contact with the old age psychiatry service she received a plethora of other treatments, including psychopharmacological treatments, occupational therapy, physiotherapy, individual supportive psychotherapy, work with her family and psychosocial interventions. She was not admitted to hospital during the 6 months after starting on M-ECT, but spent 23 weeks in hospital over the 12 month period prior to starting M-ECT.

Efficacy of ECT in late life

Abrams (1997b) states that 'if anything the response to ECT improves with the age of the patient'. Response rates are generally of the order of 70–80% or greater. Some of the relevant studies are listed in Table 5.3.

Immediate response to ECT in older people is good and there is some evidence that longer term outcome may be better than amongst comparable

Table 5.3. Response rates found in some studies of ECT in older age groups.

Study	Number of patients	Mean age	Outcome: recovered/ much improved (%)
Fraser and Glass (1980)	33	73	97
Gaspar and Samarasinghe (1982)	33	73.9	78.8
Karlinsky and Shulman (1984)	33	73.2	78.8
Godber et al. (1987)	163	76	74
Benbow (1987)	122	73	80
Rubin, Kinscherf and Wehrman (1991)	46	75.9	78[1]
Wilkinson, Anderson and Peters (1993)	43	73.9	73
Casey and Davis (1996)	18	79.5	86.3[2]

1. Wilkinson et al. (1993) compared response in under and over 65 year olds respectively in 78 patients treated with ECT. The response rate was higher in over 65s (73%) than in under 65s (54%).
2. Casey and Davis (1996) reviewed response in people aged over 75 years.

younger people. Wesson et al. (1997) followed up a group of 78 people treated with ECT (Wilkinson et al. 1993) and found that, at follow up 24–45 months after index course of ECT, increasing age was significantly associated with probability of improved prognosis. Older people do as well as, or even better than, younger people treated with ECT.

Key points

- ECT is still in use today because it is safe, effective and necessary in a small group of people who are too ill for alternative treatments or who fail to respond to alternatives.
- The response rate is of the order of 70–80% and many of the people who receive ECT will have failed to respond to other treatment regimes.
- As people respond to treatment they can take advantage of other therapies, aimed at keeping them well, and addressing any precipitating and maintaining factors in their illness.

References

Abrams, R. (1991) Electroconvulsive therapy in the medically compromised patient. *Psychiatric Clinics of North America*, **14**, 871–885.

Abrams, R. (1997a) Electroconvulsive therapy in the high-risk patient. In *Electroconvulsive Therapy*, pp. 81–113, 3rd edn. Oxford University Press, Oxford.

Abrams, R. (1997b) Efficacy of electroconvulsive therapy. In *Electroconvulsive Therapy*, pp. 11–40, 3rd edn. Oxford University Press, Oxford.

American Psychiatric Association (1990) *The Practice of Electroconvulsive Therapy: Recommendations for Treatment, Training, and Privileging.* American Psychiatric Association, Washington, DC.

Benbow, S.M. (1987) The use of electroconvulsive therapy in old age psychiatry. *International Journal of Geriatric Psychiatry*, **2**, 25–30.

Benbow, S.M. (1989) The role of electroconvulsive therapy in the treatment of depressive illness in old age. *British Journal of Psychiatry*, **155**, 147–152.

Benbow, S.M. (1991) Old age psychiatrists' views on the use of ECT. *International Journal of Geriatric Psychiatry*, **6**, 317–322.

Benbow, S.M. (1992) Is ECT useful for depression with dementia? First European Symposium on ECT, March 26–29, Graz, Austria, Abstract book, p. 3.

Benbow, S.M. (1995) Safe ECT practice in physically ill patients. In *The ECT Handbook*, edited by C.P. Freeman, pp. 26–29. Royal College of Psychiatrists, London.

Brandt, B. and Ugarriza, D.N. (1996) Electroconvulsive therapy and the elderly client. *Journal of Gerontological Nursing*, **22**, 14–20.

Burke, W.J., Rubin, E.H., Zorumski, C.F. and Wetzel, R.D. (1987) The safety of ECT in geriatric psychiatry. *Journal of the American Geriatric Society*, **35**, 516–521.

Casey, D.A. and Davis, M.H. (1996) Electroconvulsive therapy in the very old. *General Hospital Psychiatry*, **18**, 436–439.

Clarke, T.B., Coffey, C.E., Hoffman, G.W. and Weiner, R.D. (1989) Continuation therapy for depression using outpatient electroconvulsive therapy. *Convulsive Therapy*, **5**, 330–337.

Cobb, A. (1995) *Older Women and ECT*. MIND, London.

CRAG Working Group on Mental Illness (1997) *Electroconvulsive Therapy (ECT) – a Good Practice Statement*. Scottish Office.

Department of Health (1992) *Electroconvulsive Therapy England – Year Ending 31 March 1991*. Department of Health Statistics Division, London.

Department of Health (1999) *Electroconvulsive Therapy: Survey Covering the Period from January 1999 to March 1999, England*. Department of Health, Statistical Bulletin.

Dolinski, S.Y. and Zvara, D.A. (1997) Anesthetic considerations of cardiovascular risk during electroconvulsive therapy. *Convulsive Therapy*, **13**, 157–164.

Duncan, A.J., Ungvari, G.S., Russell, R.J. and Seifert, A. (1990) Maintenance ECT in very old age. *Annals of Clinical Psychiatry*, **2**, 1–6.

Fink, M. (1991) Impact of the antipsychiatry movement on the revival of electroconvulsive therapy in the United States. *Psychiatric Clinics of North America*, **4**, 793–801.

Fink, M. (1999) *Electroshock Restoring the Mind*. Oxford University Press, Oxford.

Freeman, C.P. (1995) *The ECT Handbook*. Royal College of Psychiatrists, London.

Fraser, R.M. and Glass, I.B. (1980) Unilateral and bilateral ECT in elderly patients: a comparative study. *Acta Psychiatrica Scandinavica*, **62**, 13–31.

Gaspar, D. and Samarasinghe, L.A. (1982) ECT in psychogeriatric practice – a study of risk factors, indications and outcome. *Comprehensive Psychiatry*, **23**, 170–175.

Godber, C., Rosenvinge, H., Wilkinson, D, Smithies, J. *et al.* (1987) Depression in old age: prognosis after ECT. *International Journal of Geriatric Psychiatry*, **2**, 19–24.

Karlinsky, H. and Shulman, K.T. (1984) The clinical use of electroconvulsive therapy in old age. *Journal of the American Geriatrics Society*, **32**, 183–186.

Kendell, R.E. (1981) The present status of electroconvulsive therapy. *British Journal of Psychiatry*, **139**, 265–283.

Kramer, B.A. (1987) Maintenance ECT: a survey of practice (1986) *Convulsive Therapy*, **3**, 260–268.

Lock, T. (1995) Stimulus dosing. In *The ECT Handbook*, edited by C.P. Freeman, pp. 72–87. Royal College of Psychiatrists, London.

Martin, B.A. and Bean, G.J. (1992) Competence to consent to electroconvulsive therapy. *Convulsive Therapy*, **8**, 92–102.

McCall, W.V. (1996) Asystole in electroconvulsive therapy: report of four cases. *Journal of Clinical Psychiatry*, **5**, 199–203.

Monroe, R.R. (1991) Maintenance electroconvulsive therapy. *Psychiatric Clinics of North America*, **14**, 947–960.

Olfson, M., Marcus, S., Sackeim, H.A, Thompson, J. and Pincus, H.A. *et al.* (1998) Use of ECT for the inpatient treatment of recurrent major depression. *American Journal of Psychiatry*, **155**, 22–29.

Pippard J. and Ellam, L. (1981) *Electroconvulsive Treatment in Great Britain, 1980.* Gaskell, London.

Rubin, E.H., Kinscherf, D.A. and Wehrman, S.A. (1991) Response to treatment of depression in the old and the very old. *Journal of Geriatric Psychiatry and Neurology*, **4**, 65–70.

Schwarz, T., Loewenstein, J. and Isenberg, K.E. (1995) Maintenance ECT: indications and outcome. *Convulsive Therapy*, **11**, 14–23.

Scott, A. (1995) Continuation ECT (maintenance ECT). In *The ECT Handbook*, edited by C.P. Freeman, p. 71. Royal College of Psychiatrists, London.

Stevenson, G.H. and Geoghegan, J.J. (1951) Prophylactic electroshock a five year study. *American Journal of Psychiatry*, **107**, 743–748.

Vanelle, J.-M., Loo, H., Galinowski, A, de Carvalho, W., Bourdel, M-C., Brochier, P. *et al.* (1994) Maintenance ECT in intractable manic-depressive disorders. *Convulsive Therapy*, **10**, 195–205.

Wesson, M.L., Wilkinson, A.M., Anderson, D.N. and McCracken, C. (1997) Does age predict the long-term outcome of depression treated with ECT? (A prospective study of the long-term outcome of ECT-treated depression with respect to age). *International Journal of Geriatric Psychiatry*, **12**, 45–51.

Wilkinson, A.M., Anderson, D.N. and Peters, S. (1993) Age and the effects of ECT. *International Journal of Geriatric Psychiatry*, **8**, 401–406.

Zielinski, R.J., Roose, S.P. , Devanand, D.P, Woodring, S. and Saekeim, H.A. *et al.* (1998) Cardiovascular complications of ECT in depressed patients with cardiac disease. American Journal of Psychiatry, **150**, 904–909.

The role of primary care in the assessment, diagnosis and management of depression in older people

Philip Heywood

'Miss not the discourse of the elders' Apocrypha, Ecclesiasticus, viii, 9

Introduction
Diagnosis
Assessment
Management

Introduction

Most elderly people live happy, fulfilled, independent lives until they die. As at other ages, some may have periods of physical or mental ill-health. It is a minority whose lives and lifestyles are determined by their health status. This book considers the needs of a minority of elderly patients who are depressed. However, if services are appropriate for those people with the greatest needs, they are likely to be sensitive, approachable and appropriate for those with lesser needs.

Primary care is a setting in which healthcare is provided. I shall use it to mean those community-based health services that provide preventive, primary, personal and continuing care to patients and their families; it includes responsibility for individuals and a population; it is mainly a partnership between general practice and personal community health services. However, it includes other contractor services and requires links to be managed with social services and secondary care.

It was back in the 1970s that the World Health Organization (WHO 1973) set out the reasons why primary care has such a central role in mental health care. Patients with psychosocial problems are, on average, higher users of primary care; they are consequently more likely to be known to the general practitioner and the primary health care team; those relationship can therefore be used for therapeutic interventions. There are fewer stigmas attached to general practice treatment than to psychiatric treatment. Physical and psychological problems tend to co-exist, particularly in elderly people, and they may be difficult to separate; it is easier for the general practice team to treat the many needs of the whole person. Continuing care is a feature of general practice, so that chronic or episodic illnesses can be appropriately managed long-term.

Mental health problems are extremely common in primary care, and people are no less likely to suffer from depression because they are elderly. However, it has been observed for many years that people with mental health problems are often managed poorly in general practice, as well as in other settings (Department of Health 1998, Audit Commission 2000). The findings and recommendations of the Audit Commission's report *Forget Me Not; Mental Health Services For Older People* are listed in Table 6.1. It is mainly concerned with the issues of dementia and depression in old age.

The varying standards of mental health care provision in primary care will no longer be tolerated. A new standard has been set for primary care in the National Service Framework (Department of Health 1999a). Any service user who contacts their primary health care team with a common mental health problem should have their mental health needs identified and assessed and be offered effective treatments, including referral to specialist services for further assessment, treatment and care if they require it. Clinical governance mechanisms established within the New NHS and managed within primary care groups and trusts are meant to ensure that previous poor quality services are improved or replaced (NHS Executive 1999).

Much health-care provision discriminates by age, and ageism permeates the care that is provided to elderly people. It is appropriate and necessary to respond to the special needs that advancing age brings to people; it is discriminatory to ignore those needs (it is more difficult to get an adequate story from a deaf person than a hearing person; that is not an excuse for missing depression). It is discriminatory to attribute greater disability than the needs warrant (deaf people do not have learning difficulties); and it is discriminatory to deny older patients the care that is offered to younger people merely by virtue of their age (a deaf patient is entitled to the same privacy as a younger, hearing person – although it may be difficult to provide when the patient sits in the common room of a residential home).

Couples counselling is seldom offered to octogenarians. I have done this on three occasions with considerable improvement in the marital relationship each time. I am sure that my failure to offer counselling more often to elderly

Table 6.1. The Audit Commission's report, *Forget Me Not: Mental Health Services for Older People.*

The Audit Commission's main findings:

- Only half of carers are told what the problem is, or how dementia is likely to affect their relative in the future.
- Many GPs require greater support to help effectively.
- Whilst most GPs were trained in managing depression, half had not received any specific training in managing dementia and did not use any specific tests or protocols to diagnose it.
- Older people with mental health problems could get help at an earlier stage if specialist professionals give advice and support to GPs.
- Older people with mental health problems need a thorough assessment of needs, often best carried out at home, and access to a range of services. But many do not have access to all they need, often because most of the resources for specialist mental health services come from health agencies and go on hospital and residential care.
- People who would otherwise need residential care could live at home, if provided with flexible home-based care by joint health and social services teams.

The Audit Commission's recommendations include:

- GPs and other primary care staff should provide better information, support and competent advice for users and carers.
- Mental health professionals should provide more training and support for GPs and primary care teams.
- Provision should be balanced more in favour of flexible home-based services to provide support where it is needed.
- Health and social services should work together more effectively to share information about the care of individuals and to make better use of their joint resources.
- Commissioners of health and social care should have better information about the services they provide, to whom, and how well they are working.
- Users and carers should be involved in assessments and decisions about their care.

people reflects my own ageist prejudices. The age patterns of referrals to counselling services in primary care confirm that I am not alone.

General practitioners are taught to frame their assessments in physical, psychological and social terms. Most general practitioners will be able to list the physical diagnoses, some of the psychological issues and describe the social context for many of their elderly patients. Frequently they will not integrate the three and look at the interdependence of the patients past life-history, their current physical and social conditions and their state of mental well-being.

The evidence base for primary care is the same as that for secondary care. It is therefore not my intention merely to repeat the content and messages of the other chapters. I intend to examine the features of primary care and of general practice and consider how care within that setting needs to be offered to patients. I attempt to highlight those things that are peculiar to general practice; those things that are problematic in general practice and those things that are best exemplified from general practice. For any individual patient a balance must be struck; the evidence base, often from randomized controlled trials (RCTs), must be balanced by the doctor's clinical experience, of this patient and of this setting, and by the patient's wishes (Figure 6.1).

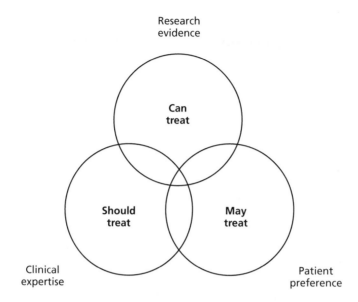

Figure 6.1 Evidence-based medicine.

Mental health care is about people. Some of those people seek help and some offer it. I am a male general practitioner who has worked in three cities in both deprived and affluent areas over the last three decades. I shall tend to use the male pronoun for the doctor and female for patients and nurses, except where the context requires otherwise.

Diagnosis

Most members of the primary health care team will be confronted by distressed, depressed elderly people. The skills and sensitivities that I describe are needed by all in the team. Nevertheless, diagnosis of physical and mental disease is still mainly undertaken by the general practitioner; therefore this is the paradigm that I have adopted in this section. Where I use the term 'doctor' or 'general practitioner' it might equally apply to nurse or psychologist when they are using diagnostic approaches in community settings.

There have been four decennial studies of morbidity in general practice. Together they provide the most representative data of morbidity in UK general practice since 1951. A large number of practices from around the country contribute. In 1991–1992 60 practices in England and Wales with more than half a million registered patients provided detailed information on 1.3 million contacts with a general practitioner (Royal College of General Practitioners 1995). Between 1981/2 and 1991/2 reduced consulting rates were recorded for mental disorders in both sexes and at all ages. (All other disease categories except 'symptoms, signs and ill-defined conditions' recorded increased consulting rates.) There is no reason to suppose a decreased prevalence of mental distress; some of the decrease may be artefactual from the way data were collected; some patients may have seen counsellors, rather than doctors and nurses. It must remain a possibility that mental illness increasingly is missed in general practice. However, within the overall decrease, consulting rates for serious mental disorders increased by more than 50%, perhaps reflecting the move into the community of people with serious chronic psychiatric illness.

There are considerable problems of defining 'cases' in general practice (Sharp and King 1989). Much psychological distress is seen at its earliest stages. The distress and morbidity is frequently transient and self-limiting; there are no agreements on how long it should be present to justify case-ness. Each psychiatric disorder lies along a continuum from 'normality' to 'extremity'; the degree of distress or disability required to induce case-ness is not agreed; each doctor makes his own judgements. The availability of appropriate interventions may determine the doctor's willingness to make a diagnosis.

With all ages of patients, psychological diagnoses are missed in general practice; for elderly patients most often we miss depression and dementia. Some factors have been identified as contributing to failure to make such diagnoses in hospital; it is likely that similar factors operate in primary care. The patient may provide no obvious cues; the doctor may fail to pick up cues; patients may lack the privacy to disclose (this is important in residential settings); having found organic disorder the doctor may look no further for psychological illness; even when a psychological disorder is suspected the doctor may lack the confidence to pursue the assessment (Goldberg 1985).

Higgs (1994, 1999) presents a more challenging and perhaps more likely possibility. He questions how often the patient is the only depressed person in the doctor–patient encounter; he wonders how often our 'deafness' to other people's depression arises from our own depression; he questions whether the motivation to medicine carries a specific risk to depression and whether we are unable to look after our own mental well-being.

Many people feel depressed; a few suffer from a depressive illness. The distinction is important because the interventions may differ; but both must be recognized and treated. The patient with depressive illness is no more worthy of care than the patient with depressed mood. We must respond to the patient's distress, not to the diagnostic label which we apply for our benefit.

Although most elderly people live happy, fulfilled, independent lives, many others are lonely, isolated, dependent, tired, and may have restricted mobility, visual handicap or partial hearing; the diseases of ageing may have brought physical limitation or handicap; many take medication. Any of these factors may be a cause of depression or may accompany depression. But none, of itself, is depression. Depression may be mainly a patient's response to circumstances, or may arise without obvious precipitants. However, the first episode of an endogenous depression in old age is unusual. Elderly people are at risk for many reasons.

Depression is a concomitant of some other diseases that are common in old age, whether as an adjustment disorder or intrinsic to the physical disease. Early dementia and Parkinson's disease may both induce depression. The differentiation of dementia and depression can be particularly difficult. Significant memory loss may be experienced by some elderly people with moderate depression; and depression can coexist with dementia. Stroke, malignant disease, myocardial infarction, chronic obstructive airways disease and hypothyroidism seem to be especially depressing conditions.

There is often dis-empowerment as a consequence of the changes of age. These days fewer people reach old age before they retire; nevertheless, the loss of role that accompanies retirement can be stressful for the retired, but can also depress the spouse because of the imposed change of life-style and the increased time spent with each other. Increasing dependence on others can further move the patient's locus of control. There are common losses associated with ageing some of which are acute, and some gradual. There may be loss of mobility, of special senses, of continence, of independence, of residence with consequent distancing of friends and neighbours; there may be bereavement, mutilating surgery, rejection and ultimately dying.

Some elderly patients, after a major loss, choose not to grieve. It is as if they feel it is not worth the work that will be necessary. They would rather remain unchanged until their own death. If this comes quickly there is no problem; if they survive for years, their depression can become manifest much later. A particularly distressing and common situation can occur when an elderly woman lives with her daughter and son-in-law. Relationships may be good, neutral or poor. However, if the son-in-law dies before the mother, the two women can have difficulty sharing their grief. The mother feels guilty, and the daughter may feel angry, at the son-in-laws 'untimely' death and the mother's 'untimely' survival.

It may also be a time of reflection. The elderly people of today were young adults during the war. Some were in the forces; others may have come to UK as refugees. They may have experienced violence and hardship that has been suppressed in memory for most of a lifetime. Others may have lifelong suppressed memories of childhood abuse, physical or sexual. Some elderly people find these distant feelings and hazy memories start to surface and lead to depression and despair. They usually have had no practice at talking about the events, and need a gentle and supportive doctor who will help, encourage and allow them to explore such memories, without any pressure to reveal those things that the patient does not wish.

However, if we recognize those patients who apparently accord with the diagnostic features of major depression in DSM-IV (American Psychiatric Association 1996), how many are depressed? In reaching a diagnosis of depression it is usual to give weight to the physical symptoms that accompany the mood changes. Without knowing the prevalence of those symptoms in an elderly population, and therefore their sensitivity and specificity for depression, it is impossible to be confident about the diagnosis. Sleep disturbance, weight loss, weight gain and anorexia may all accompany ageing, the diseases of ageing and medications used for diseases of ageing. How, then, can we be sure when they are indicative of depression?

On the other hand, if we only treat patients who accord to DSM-IV criteria, we will leave many with their distress. Experience in general practice shows that we must be much more eclectic in our approach to our ageing patients, lest we miss their distress and opportunities to relieve it.

Since psychological distress and psychiatric diagnoses are frequently missed, the assessment of elderly people's mental health must improve. General practice is conventionally considered the gateway to other services, therefore improvement is most necessary in primary care. The barriers must be acknowledged and overcome. Some such barriers are general to all patients, some are specific to elderly people.

Assessment

To recognize the distress of our depressed patients we must learn to listen, to hear, to feel and to respond.

The public view of the medical encounter is that the patient sets out the health problem and the general practitioner makes a diagnosis and plans treatment. Such an account provides an insufficient description of the roles of both parties. In reality the patient may feel distress which she cannot articulate. She may suspect the cause of her distress, but be diffident to talk about it (whether the suspicion is correct or not). She may believe her distress is, in some way, normal and not feel any need to consult about it, but be encouraged to consult by someone else.

In response to the arrival of a patient, the doctor is taught to 'take a history'. Although there items of information that the doctor may need for his purposes, 'taking' is an inappropriate verb to describe the process. The patient has a story to tell. The doctor needs to hear that story. To enable the patient to tell the story the doctor needs to be interested. It is not sufficient to feign interest, with polished social skills; the doctor needs to be interested and inquisitive to know what the patient has to say. And he must recognize how she makes him feel. Moods and emotions can be infectious; the doctor must learn to feel the patient's condition as well as to hear it. But feeling patients' feelings carries a cost. As doctors and nurses in primary care we deal with patients' emotional problems without external supervision. No psychologist, counsellor, psychotherapist or social worker would consider such a risky approach to caring for other people's emotional problems. We must learn to discuss these patients with each other to protect the patients and to protect ourselves emotionally.

Medical interviewing is based on the assumption that the patient can tell the doctor what concerns her, answer what the doctor asks her and disclose what the doctor needs to know from her. It is arrogant to assume that she wants to tell her story to the doctor, or that she is able to tell the doctor. She may fear telling the doctor. Some of the things that patients wish to talk about are difficult to voice. The general practitioner's job is to enable patients to develop a language to express their thoughts and feelings and articulate their distress. Sometimes patients are trying to say things that they have never been able to say before.

The first stage of medical interviewing is to greet the patient and put them at their ease. We know that patients, particularly elderly patients, find it difficult to be critical of their general practitioner; they are more disposed to express satisfaction and to be compliant, even when dissatisfied (Department of Health 1999b). There is therefore a major onus on the doctor to consider what will make communication easiest for each individual patient. Some patients choose to attend the surgery, where it may be easier to maintain privacy; but the doctor will need to work hard to ensure that the patient does not feel the pressure of time, particularly if his consultations are already running late. Many elderly patients are seen in their homes. They have the advantage of being on their own territory; but it may be difficult to ensure there is privacy when *the patient* requires it. The spouse or a carer may habitually be part of the consultation with the patient's consent; it can be difficult to appropriately change this later when the patient needs a private discussion.

Privacy can be even more difficult for patients in residential settings. The time taken to move someone from a sitting room to a private room may take longer that the consultation itself. It can be difficult to exclude the professional carers, particularly when it is necessary; such as when an elderly person wishes to disclose some abuse within the home.

If the patient is deaf or visually handicapped there may be further problems for confidentiality. A blind patient needs to be told explicitly who is present at the consultation, and still informed if only the doctor is attending. Deaf patients need to hear the doctor; but the doctor must find a setting to ensure that others do not overhear his words. In all settings privacy extends beyond the contact with the patient. Information that is revealed to others after the consultation should be released only with the patient's explicit consent. If the patient sees that the doctor makes these efforts while they are together, she is more likely to trust him with more sensitive things later.

Patients invite the doctor into their lives when the doctor shows genuine interest in that life, sharing the highs and the lows and the significant moments – significant to the patient. Diagnosis is not a process of following a track to a single label; it is an attempt to paint a rich picture of a whole person, with a history and a life-long set of relationships that give meaning to today's distress. There is no single tag, label or diagnosis. She is not depressed merely because her husband has died. Her loss only has meaning when the nature of the previous life is described. Has she lost a supportive life companion; if so, how was he supportive, so what is now missing? Has she lost 50 years of being abused; if so, whom can she now tell? Has she lost the focus of her life as a carer? And within each of those there are further layers of depth and of meaning.

The first requirement of the health professional is therefore an ability to listen. Most of us believe that we are good at listening. But patients tell us otherwise. This account by an adult (but not elderly) ex-patient is a glowing account of good care, but is thereby a strong indictment of the care he had previously received (Case History 6.1).

If the environment, the confidentiality and the general practitioner's skills

Case History 6.1

'Only once in 15 years of psychiatric intervention, and at the age of 36, was I able to find someone who was willing to listen . . . This nurse actually found time to listen to my experiences and feelings. She always made me feel welcome, and would make arrangements so we would not be disturbed. She would switch off her bleeper and take her phone off the hook, and sometimes, as there were people outside her room, she would close the blinds. These actions would make me feel at ease . . . She told me that what we said was confidential, but that there were some exceptions, so I could decide what to reveal . . . Sometimes when I was describing what happened to me she would tell me that it was hurting her and she needed a break. At last, I had found someone who recognized the pain that I was feeling.' (Romme and Escher 1993).

are managed, the doctor's listening can be augmented by the strategies described in Chapters 2 and 7. The diagnostic features are no different in primary care than elsewhere, and the checklists to identify depression and dementia as useful as in other settings.

Management

The evidence used to support appropriate management must be combined from two sources. However, there is little advice how to achieve that. One source is the population approach of evidence-based medicine (Sackett *et al.* 1997) and the other is the individual focus of a narrative-based approach (Balint 1986, Greenhalgh 1998).

Evidence-based medicine is the conscientious and judicious use of current best evidence from clinical care research in the management of individual patients. This book considers the evidence base that should underpin patient care. The evidence base for primary care is the same as that for secondary care. Therefore the information on management contained in other chapters is of relevance to patients in community settings. There are no problems with the evidence; however, there may be difficulties in trying to apply the evidence in community settings.

It has been shown that therapeutic interventions in general practice are as likely to be based on evidence as those in a general medical, hospital setting (Gill *et al.* 1996, Ellis *et al.* 1995). Nevertheless, the application of the evidence base in general practice requires two qualifications. One relates to the evidence, and one relates to the setting; these are listed in Table 6.2.

Much of general practice consists of medicine that combines science with art, sociology, mythology or pastoral care. These aspects of care must be incorporated into an appropriate paradigm of evidence-based practice rather than

Table 6.2. Issues in applying research-based evidence in primary care.

The research evidence:

- Evidence-based medicine requires that data generated from populations are applied to individuals. How well represented was *this* patient in the studies?
- There are many outcomes of randomised controlled trials (RCT)—speed of recovery; time to relapse; level of side-effects; acceptability to patients; effect on usage of concurrent therapies; etc. Which, if any, outcomes are paramount; and are they paramount for *this* patient?
- RCTs will not necessarily indicate the most cost-effective current treatment for general practice.
- RCT evidence has been presented with the value of a 'gold standard'; perhaps, since it is likely to be altered by tomorrow's experience, it has more the value of a 'coffee future'!
- Many interventions have been originally assessed within secondary care; how appropriate is that for subsequent application in the community?

The primary care setting:

- Patients present in general practice with multiple and/or ill-defined problems.
- It may be difficult to allocate a specific diagnosis to a symptom.
- A specific diagnosis may not be reached within a single consultation.
- There are patients in whom the pathology is neither clear nor relevant to the patient's problem.
- The presence of any pathology is usually not proven by investigations.
- Consultations may be triggered by a large number of circumstances (e.g. certification, external pressure), rather than a clinical event.
- Diagnoses and interventions are usually multiple, with physical, psychological and social elements.
- There is pressure to record a medical diagnosis to justify treatment (Howie 1972).
- Secondary diagnoses may not be recorded in GP records, and social problems may not be mentioned.

that determined solely by clinical trial. Linked to this, is the search for appropriateness of the methods used to provide the evidence. For general practice, and possibly in other settings too, the most important evidence may be found in developing alternative methodologies which complement conclusions from RCTs.

Whilst the evidence base may define what is desirable, the local configuration of services may dictate what is possible.

Team care is much more relevant to management than to diagnosis for elderly patients with mental health problems. The professionals who are acknowledged as members of the primary health care team vary from place to place. General practitioners, community/district nurses, health visitors, and practice nurses are usually counted in; the practice's administrative staff may also be included. Practice-based counsellors and psychologists are often included, but excluded if not practice-based. The inclusion of community psychiatric nurses, social workers and psychiatric social workers is very variable. Mental health professionals tend to cluster together in the larger training practices, and there is no relationship between their distribution and the age of the practice population (Kendrick *et al.* 1993).

If patients are to benefit maximally, all the involved professionals need to exchange information and share decision-making. The actual membership of the team is less important than the systems the team members set up to communicate between themselves, and with other relevant groups, such as the community psychiatric team and the local social work team.

However, team care can present a problem for patients, perhaps worse for elderly people. It may not be easy to relate to a team. If many different health workers are each involved the patient can become confused; if a single (key) worker is chosen, ways must be found to involve the patient in choosing which person in the team that should be. This is relevant for patients from minority ethnic backgrounds; cultural sensitivity is particularly necessary for the humane treatment of elders. Too often patients are given the worker whom the team feels is most appropriate.

Some patients are wholly managed in primary care, some in secondary care and some jointly. Most reach secondary care through referral, although patients who present as psychiatric emergencies often reach secondary care without seeing a general practitioner. Most people in secondary care, and many in primary care, fail to understand the many reasons why patients are referred. In fact, seven conditions must be met if the general practitioner is to manage the patient without referral somewhere (not necessarily to secondary care). These conditions are listed in Figure 6.2.

If the referring doctor is clear why they have made the referral, and if they include this information in the referral letter (or other referral communication) the patient is much more likely to receive the services they require from secondary care. But in many places there has been no agreement between psychiatrists and general practitioners what is the essential information to exchange. The opinions of one groups of psychiatrists and general practitioners is represented in Table 6.3. Although there is some uncertainly about the contents for the initial referral letter and for the response from the specialist services, there is even more problem with the continuing communication. Each district must set up robust systems so that information can be shared about patients with mental health problems who are treated simultaneously in primary and secondary care. The National Service Framework prescribes a written care plan for service users on the Care Programme Approach, but it should be provided for all patients so that the patient, their carers and the health care providers all understand the management that has been planned. Hence a structural approach to assessment, diagnosis and management can improve the experience of an elderly patient with a mental health problem. The real future challenge is to practice preventive mental health.

Key points

- Distressed elderly patients should have the causes of their distress identified, their mental health needs assessed and be offered effective treatments.
- For most patients, this can be provided by the primary health care team.
- If the patient requires it, they should be referred to specialist services for further assessment, treatment and care.
- This chapter has tried to identify some of the barriers to successfully achieving these aims in primary care.

1. Can an adequate level of diagnosis be achieved?

    ↓

    Yes   → No → Refer

    ↓

2. Can appropriate management/therapy be provided?

    ↓

    Yes   → No → Refer

    ↓

3. Is the prognosis better at home?

    ↓

    Yes   → No → Refer

    ↓

4. Have the carers the capacity to cope?

    ↓

    Yes   → No → Refer

    ↓

5. Has the patient the capacity to cope?

    ↓

    Yes   → No → Refer

    ↓

6. Are the home circumstances suitable?

    ↓

    Yes   → No → Refer

    ↓

7. Has the doctor the capacity to cope?

    ↓

    Yes   → No → Refer

    ↓

MANAGE IN PRIMARY CARE

Figure 6.2 Seven conditions to be met to avoid referral.

Table 6.3. Key items requested to be included in letters between psychiatrists and general practitioners (Pullen and Yellowlees 1985).

Items requested by 120 psychiatrists in referral letters from general practitioners:	
Main symptom/problem	100%
Reason for referral	88%
Psychiatric history	72%
Medication	62%
Family history	37%
Items requested by 120 general practitioners in replies from psychiatrists:	
Follow up	95%
Treatment	92%
Diagnosis	88%
Concise explanation	60%
Prognosis	23%

References

American Psychiatric Association (1996) *Diagnostic and Statistical Manual of Mental Disorders: Primary Care Version*, 1st edn. American Psychiatric Association, Washington, DC.

Audit Commission (2000) *Forget Me Not: Mental Health Services for Older People*. Audit Commission Publications, London.

Balint, M. (1986) *The Doctor, his Patient and the Illness*, 2nd edn. Churchill Livingstone, Edinburgh.

Department of Health (1998) *Modernising Mental Health Services: Safe, Sound and Supportive*, pp. 24–31. Department of Health, London.

Department of Health (1999a) *National Service Framework for Mental Health*. Department of Health, London.

Department of Health (1999b) *Quality and Performance in the New NHS; National Surveys of NHS Patients: General Practice 1998*. Department of Health, London.

Ellis, J., Mulligan, I., Rowe, J. and Sackett, D. (1995) Inpatient general medicine is evidence based. *Lancet*, **346**, 407–410.

Gill, P. , Dowell, A.C., Neal, R.D., Smith, N., Heywood, P. L. and Wilson, A. (1996) Evidence based general practice – a retrospective study of interventions in one training practice. *British Medical Journal*, **312**, 819–821.

Goldberg, D. (1985) Identifying psychiatric illness among general medical patients. *British Medical Journal*, **291**, 161–162.

Greenhalgh, T. (1998) Narrative based medicine in an evidence based world. In *Narrative Based Medicine*, edited by T. Greenhalgh and B. Hurwitz pp. 247–265. BMJ Books, London.

Higgs, R. (1994) Doctors in crisis: creating a strategy for mental health in health care work. *Journal of the Royal College of Physicians of London*, **28**, 538–540.

Higgs, R. (1999) Depression in general practice. In *General Practice and Ethics*, edited by C. Dowrick and L. Frith, pp. 134–149. Routledge, London.

Howie, J.G.R. (1972) Diagnosis: The Achilles heel. *Journal of the Royal College of General Practitioners*, **22**, 310.

Kendrick, T., Sibbald, B., Addington-Hall, J., Brenneman, D. and Freeling, P. (1993) Distribution of mental health professionals working on site in English and Welsh general practices. *British Medical Journal*, **307**, 544–546.

NHS Executive (1999) *National Clinical Governance: Quality in the New NHS*. HSC 1999/065. Department of Health, London.

Pullen, I. and Yellowlees, A. (1985) Is communication improving between general practitioners and psychiatrists. *British Medical Journal*, **290**, 31–33.

Romme, M. and Escher, S. (1993) *Accepting Voices*, p. 141. MIND, London.

Royal College of General Practitioners, Office of Population Censuses and Surveys, Department of Health (1995) *Morbidity Statistics from General Practice. Fourth National Study 1991–1992*, pp. 69–71. HMSO, London.

Sackett, D.L., Richardson, W.S., Rosenberg, W. and Haynes, R.B. (1997) *Evidence-Based Medicine. How to Practice and Teach EBM*. Churchill Livingstone, London.

Sharp, D.J. and King, M.B. (1989) Classification of psychosocial disturbance in general practice. *Journal of the Royal College of General Practitioners*, **39**, 356–358.

WHO (1973) *Psychiatry and Primary Medical Care*. WHO Regional Office for Europe, Copenhagen.

Depression in physically ill older patients

Graham Mulley

Introduction

It should be easy to diagnose and treat depression in physically ill older people. The manifestations of depressive illness are well known and there are effective treatments, which are readily available. In practice, things are not straightforward. Even if physicians discern that patients are depressed, they may be uncertain whether to prescribe drugs (and if so, which ones, in what dosage and for how long) and when and if to refer to a consultant in old age psychiatry.

In this chapter I will explain why depression is so important in elderly medical patients, examine the relationship between depression and physical illness and explore the reasons why depression is under-diagnosed. I will then suggest ways in which its recognition can be improved. Looking at published evidence, I will outline treatments of depression and suggest how we might improve clinical practice. Finally, I will offer directions for future research.

Why is depression important in sick older people?

Depression is the commonest psychiatric condition in medical inpatients. Published studies give different rates for its prevalence. In particular there are variations in:

- the populations sampled;
- the diagnostic tools used; and
- the cut-off points used to determine the severity of depression.

In general medical wards, about a third of patients will have symptoms of depression and a quarter will have a depression syndrome. The figures are higher on geriatric wards. Not only is depression unpleasant for the patient, but it causes distress to the family and presents challenges to the ward staff. Depression is very important because it is associated with:

- Increased mortality: depressed patients have a higher mortality rate than their age- and sex-matched controls. The death rate is three times greater in depressed men and twice as high in women compared with controls (Burell *et al.* 1991). Most of these deaths are due to acute medical illnesses, particularly stroke and myocardial infarction.
- Greater morbidity: depression worsens the prognosis of the co-existing physical illness. (This is partly due to reduced activity.)
- Reduced activity: depressed patients are less able to do everyday activities. This reduction in function adds to the complexity of rehabilitation, the main aims of which are to optimize function and well-being.
- Reduced compliance: older people who are depressed are less likely to continue to take their medication. This includes antidepressant medication. Medical relapses and re-admission are therefore more likely. Depression is a reason for non-attendance at clinics and refusal to have investigations.
- A greater risk of suicide: although older people are no more likely to be depressed than those in middle life, they more commonly take their lives.
- Prolonged length of hospital stay.
- Increased likelihood of going into institutional care: as treatment can improve outcome, the early detection and appropriate treatment of depression is supremely important.

The relationships between depression and physical illness

Medically ill old people are often depressed but the depression is not necessarily the result of their physical condition.

Depression may present with somatic symptoms

Some patients somatize their depressive illness. They may present with general aches and pains, a variety of bowel symptoms or sleep disturbance.

Depression can be important in the genesis of some physical conditions

Once other risk factors have been included, myocardial infarction is 4–5 times more common in men with depression. There is also an increased risk of myocardial infarction in depressed women. The risk is greater in more severe depression.

Depression is also associated with a reduction of bone density in the hip and lumbar spine. The mechanisms are unclear, though hypercorticolism and lowered osteocalin concentrations may be contributory (Dinan 1999).

The treatment of depression can cause physical problems

Side-effects of tricyclic antidepressants include postural hypotension (especially in patients with heart failure), which can result in falls and fractures. They also cause cardiac rhythm disturbances: they prolong the QT interval and cause dysrhythmias in those who already have heart conduction disorders. Selective serotonin uptake inhibitors can cause nausea, diarrhoea and headache; some of them alter the pharmacokinetics of drugs such as warfarin and calcium channel blockers. They can cause cardiac dysrhythmias if taken in overdose.

Depression may antedate or reflect serious pathology

In a survey of 209 medically ill patients in hospital, 29% were found to be depressed. Half of them dated the onset of their depression to at least 6 months before their admission (Hammond et al. 1993). There are anecdotal reports of unexplained depression in people who are later found to have underlying cancer (particularly bronchial and pancreatic cancer).

Physical illness can cause depression

We will examine some specific conditions and consider the implications for other organic diseases.

(A) CHRONIC OBSTRUCTIVE PULMONARY DISEASE (COPD)

It is difficult to determine which symptoms are related to the chronic obstructive pulmonary disease (COPD) and which to depression: tiredness, lethargy and altered libido occur in both. In one study, depression occurred in over

40% of people with COPD and was particularly common in those who were disabled. The diagnosis is easily overlooked: the doctor may attribute the patient's difficulty in doing daily living activities and reduced social participation solely to the COPD (Yohannes *et al.* 1998).

(B) STROKE

Depression occurs in about 50% of stroke patients who survive to 6 months. In half of these, there is major depression. Again, the diagnosis is not always easy: emotionalism (the patient crying or sometimes laughing easily, usually in the context of symptom discussion, sadness or sentimentality) may easily be mistaken for depression (Mulley and House 1995). Interestingly, emotionalism can respond to antidepressant medication, even in the absence of depressive illness. Depression after stroke influences outcomes: depressed patients do not rehabilitate successfully. They may be perceived as being 'difficult' or poorly motivated. The informal caregivers of stroke patients are sometimes under strain and may themselves be depressed.

(C) CANCER

Over a third of cancer patients develop psychological morbidity within 2 years of the diagnosis (Maguire and Howell 1995). In one survey, a quarter of consecutively admitted cancer patients on an oncology ward had affective disorders. In only half of them was the depression recognized. The prevalence of depression in cancer increases with more serious illness.

DEPRESSION MAY COMPLICATE PHYSICAL ILLNESS BY A REACTION TO IT OR BE ASSOCIATED WITH ORGANIC DISEASE

Studies of depression in arthritis, diabetes mellitus, after hip fracture and in elderly surgical patients have added to our understanding of depression complicating physical illness. As might be expected, depression is commoner in people:

- with chronic or severe pain;
- who are disfigured or disabled;
- whose condition is progressive; and
- who have unpleasant investigations or treatment.

However, it is difficult to predict which patients are at particular risk: some cope magnificently in the face of severe disability, others are profoundly distressed by apparently minor impairments or minimal disabilities.

DEPRESSION MAY BE A RESULT OF DRUG THERAPY FOR PHYSICAL DISEASE

It is vital to take a detailed drug history as several drugs can cause depression. The older anti-hypertensive drugs such as reserpine and methyl dopa are rarely used now, but beta blockers and nifedipine can cause depression.

Steroids are another recognized cause. Centrally acting drugs which might be incriminated include barbiturates, benzodiazepines and phenothiazines.

Some cancer patients date the onset of their depressive symptoms to a few hours after the onset of treatment with chemotherapy or deep X-ray treatment.

DEPRESSION AND PHYSICAL ILLNESS MAY COINCIDE

The person who has been bereaved or who has recurrent episodes of depression may develop on unrelated medical problem which necessitates admission to hospital. For others, coming into hospital (with its implications for loss of control and privacy) may be a depressing experience.

Why is depression under-recognized in medically ill older people?

The patient

If doctors make it clear that they are actively listening to the patient's concerns and if they ask open question ('how are you?', 'what is troubling you?') most patients will reveal their main concerns in the next 4–5 minutes. The skilled clinician will not interrupt but may offer gentle prompts – 'anything else?', 'any other problems? – it does not matter if it is something minor'. During this vital part of the clinical encounter, many patients not only reveal their symptoms, but may suggest possible causes or diagnoses and may express underlying anxieties ('Is it cancer? That is what happened to my father when he was my age'). The secret is not to interrupt – to do so may stop the patient telling you what is wrong and what is worrying them.

Yet even in the presence of a sympathetic, receptive, unhurried and holistic clinician, few older people will say that they are depressed. Why?

Some may feel that depression is a normal feature of ageing or illness. Others may be ashamed, perhaps believing that to be depressed is a sign of weakness, a lack of moral fibre. The lack of privacy on a ward may inhibit expression of very personal melancholic feelings. A few may fear the prospect of being sent to a psychiatrist, of being considered 'mad'. They may believe that psychological symptoms will be of no interest to the physician. Even if they were, the patient might prefer the doctor to focus on physical complaints and not be diverted. This may be particularly so in cancer patients, who might worry that time spent on psychological aspects mean that less attention will be paid to their physical survival.

Some depressed patients may not realize that depression can be alleviated. Others may not realize that they are depressed. Therefore in many cases, depression remains hidden. In others, it may find expression in anxiety, irritability, anger or poor memory. Some patients, perhaps fearful of the stigma of psychiatric illness, will legitimize their depression by somatization. They complain of a range of physical symptoms (especially pains in the head or gastro-intestinal symptoms) for which no evidence can be found on examination or investigation.

The clinical manifestations of depression can be classified as follows (Devinsky 1992):

- **affective** – anhedonia, sadness, anxiety, irritability;
- **cognitive** – guilt, hopelessness, impaired concentration, forgetfulness;
- **somatic** – pain, gastro-intestinal symptoms;
- **psychotic** – delusions and hallucinations; and
- **vegetative** – altered sleep and appetite, fatigue, constipation, decreased libido, psychomotor retardation.

In ill older people, the vegetative (or biological) features which might help the doctor to diagnose depression are often less useful. These include:

(a) Insomnia: the architecture of sleep usually changes with age. Older people sleep less at night and tend to nap in the day. Nocturnal sleep is more broken. Sleep may be disturbed by leg cramp, nocturia or dyspnoea. Early morning wakening is not uncommon.

(b) Fatigue: tiredness may be the result of heart failure, anaemia or chronic airways disease. Medications can make people feel fatigued, e.g. beta blockers and sedatives. The patient may be a caregiver for an elderly spouse and the hard work sometimes involved in caring can cause weariness.

(c) Anorexia: hospital food is not always appetising or well presented. It may be offered at times when the patient does not feel like eating. Those who are constipated often lose their appetite, as do people on inappropriate doses of digoxin.

(d) Constipation: many inpatients are constipated. Some have a long history which relates to a diet low in fruit, vegetables, cereals or wholemeal bread. Long-term laxative ingestion is associated with sluggish bowels. Bowel transit time is slower in anyone who is immobile. Slowed transit time is common in parkinsonism – even if the patient remains mobile. Many drugs constipate. The change of routine and diet on coming into hospital often adds to this problem.

(e) Weight loss: many people gradually lose weight during normal ageing. People living alone – particularly bereaved old men – may not bother to cook. Eating alone may mean that dietary intake is suboptimal. Cancer and heart disease can cause cachexia. Those who are blind or paralysed may have difficulty getting enough to eat on a busy understaffed ward. On the other hand, weight loss may be desirable – loss of fluid in the successful treatment of congestive cardiac failure, for example.

(f) Altered facial expression: an inexpressive face is a feature of parkinsonism. People whose dentures have not been brought into hospital may feel embarrassed to be seen without them. They may smile less or try to cover their mouths with their hands. Ptosis can be a feature of normal ageing.

(g) Reduced libido – though many older people maintain interest in and enthusiasm for sexual expression, others feel that the flames of passion dwindle with age. Many have little opportunity – especially those who are bereaved or whose loved ones are in care. In women, vaginal dryness may be associated with dyspareunia. In men, arterial or neurological impairments are causes of erectile dysfunction, as are many drugs.

(h) Retardation: physical slowing is common in many very old people. Gait becomes slower and activities take longer – especially if there is arthritis, stroke or parkinsonism.

Not only are the biological signposts to depression less helpful, but some of the affective and cognitive manifestations may also be of limited diagnostic value including:

(a) Anhedonia: a core feature of clinical depression is the reduced ability to experience pleasure. But the visually impaired person may no longer be able to enjoy books, the patient with stroke may be denied the pleasure of country walks, the musician with arthritic hands may not now be able to play the piano and the deaf person may not enjoy conversation at parties.

(b) Declining memory: it is common for older people who are not depressed or demented to have memory difficulties – especially retrieving people's names and information stored in the short-term memory.

Doctors and nurses

Whereas all doctors specializing in the psychiatry of old age have a postgraduate grounding in general medicine, few physicians have clinical experience in psychiatry. Similarly, most nurses on medical wards for older people have not received training in psychiatric nursing. Medical staff may therefore not feel competent or confident in assessing depressed patients. Some may have negative notions about psychiatric conditions and limit their attention to physical disease. A doctor's discomfiture with psychological medicine may be transmitted to the patient, who may therefore not divulge details of their mental state.

In an essay on the psychological care of patients with cancer, Maguire and Howell (1995) describe shortcomings in doctors' responses to depression. (These may also occur when doctors talk to other physically ill patients who do not have cancer.) These include:

- **deflection** – switching the subject;
- **selectivity** – the patient talks of physical and psychological concerns, but the doctor selectively focuses on the physical aspects;
- **avoidance** – the doctor may deliberately avoid asking a woman how she feels about losing a breast;
- **premature reassurance** – 'everything will be alright';
- **false reassurance** – pretending that the situation is better than it is, thus blocking the opportunity for further discussion;

- **jollying** the patient along; and
- **passing the buck** – hoping that a more senior doctor will sort out the depressive aspects of patient care.

Lack of training, not possessing the skills to deal with depression, not having enough time, being fearful of unleashing anger or despair all play a part in clinicians using these distancing or avoiding tactics.

How to improve the recognition of depression in medically ill patients

Given the prevalence and importance of depression, it is important to make the diagnosis and to do so at the earliest opportunity. This could be achieved in a number of ways:

The clinical history

A section in the medical record on psychological health should be mandatory. In practice, there is a low acknowledgement of depression in case notes. The doctor should enquire about a family history of depression and the previous use of ECT or antidepressant drugs.

Patients should be gently asked about loss of relish for life, lack of well-being, whether they have dark thoughts or a heavy heart, if they feel like crying or believe that it is not worth continuing. Asking tactfully about suicidal intent rarely seems to cause distress to older patients.

(A) PHYSICAL SIGNS

Though some depressed patients may have a facade of cheerfulness (and their close relatives may not consider the possibility of depression), others look sad. They may avoid eye contact, show few signs of animation, appear defeated or desolate. Some cry when asked about their mood. They may not initiate conversation, or reply to questions in monosyllables.

Some depressed old people will be irritable, others anxious or angry. Others seem to emanate an aura of gloom or heaviness, which the astute clinician may discern. In all these instances, the doctor should consider that the patient could be depressed.

(B) OBSERVATIONS BY THE REHABILITATION TEAM

Therapists may identify depression during individual treatment sessions or on a pre-discharge home visit (House and Ebrahim 1996). The failure of a patient to rehabilitate successfully should always raise the possibility of depression. On many medical wards for older people, nurses do not recognize depression, they sometimes mistake it for delirium or dementia (Bowler *et al.* 1994).

If they are trained in psychological aspects of health and encouraged by doctors to report on mood problems on ward rounds and at case conferences, nurses can detect those who are depressed. Refusal of medication for physical illness may be a sign of depression. It is important to ask the family – especially in stroke or other conditions where it may not be easy to distinguish depressive symptomatology from effects of the disease.

(C) AT-RISK PATIENTS

Particular attention should be given to those who are at a greater risk of depression: patients who are bereaved, lonely, who have suffered family disharmony; those with painful, progressive, dehabilitating medical conditions; those with vascular dementia, who at times have insight into their mental deterioration.

In practice, relying on clinical observations is often unsuccessful in identifying those who are depressed.

The use of screening tools

Geriatricians often use the abbreviated mental test score to identify patients with cognitive impairment. The use of screening tests for depression is less widespread. Why is this? Firstly there is a bewildering array of tests designed to identify the presence or severity of depression. Some take a long time to administer (and therefore are prone to a low response rate), others are short (but may be less sensitive). Some are self-completed, others filled in by an interviewer (who needs special training for certain tests). The tests may be structured or semi-structured. Some are written, others processed by computer. Secondly, many old people are unable to comply with such questionnaires. Those with impaired vision and hearing, dysarthria or dysphasia or cognitive problems, and those who are physically ill simply cannot cope with screening questionnaires or soon become fatigued. Thirdly, the scales may not be appropriate for the older patient. Many were developed for use in younger people. They give points for physical symptoms (so ill old people who are not depressed score highly) and may not allow for the different scores that older people register on mood scales. Fourthly, the reliance on screening tools may mean that doctors might miss the subtle or atypical features of depression in old age (e.g. agitation, anger, irritability). Nonetheless, screening tests can be helpful – especially if they are brief, easy to administer, sensitive and relevant. Some older people may be more likely to admit to sadness and dysphoria on self-rating scales than during conventional history-taking. A critique of all the available tools is beyond the scope of this chapter, but a consideration of some of them might be helpful.

(A) GERIATRIC MENTAL STATE (GMS)

This gives a cross-sectional picture of the patient's mental state giving diagnoses across a broad spectrum of psychiatric illnesses. It minimizes the attribution of depression to symptoms caused by physical illness. The GMS examines the mental state in the 4 weeks before the interview. A semi-structured interview takes 20–30 minutes to administer. The data from questionnaire are fed into a laptop computer. There is a high inter-rater reliability. As well as giving diagnostic categories, it also provides measures of severity (0 = absent, 5 = severe).

Though the GMS is one of the few tests validated for use in older people, it needs a trained interviewer, is time-consuming and is perhaps too cumbersome to be used routinely as a screening test on geriatric wards.

(B) THE CENTER FOR EPIDEMIOLOGICAL STUDIES DEPRESSION STATE (CES-D)

The original version has been widely used in studies of late-life depression. However, the time taken to complete it upsets some patients. Older people are less likely than younger ones to say that they feel sad or that people are unfriendly.

A 10–item scale (which takes 2 minutes to administer) is less stressful to the patient and has high levels of sensitivity and specificity (Irwin et al. 1999).

(C) THE HOSPITAL ANXIETY AND DEPRESSION SCALE (HAD)

This scale is limited to anxiety and depression (each of which is scored separately). It was designed to detect these conditions in medical patients. A self-assessment scale, it is brief, acceptable and useful in outpatient clinics. It can be used to record a patient's progress. However, in a study of patients on a medical ward for older people, the HAD scale lacked sensitivity and specificity. Many of those who scored highly on the anxiety scores were clearly depressed. As the HAD misses many cases and gives false positives in medically ill old people, it cannot be recommended for case-finding on elderly care wards (Davies et al. 1993).

(D) THE GERIATRIC DEPRESSION SCALE (GDS)

This screening test, which detects depression likely to benefit from treatment, is recommended by the British Geriatrics Society and the Royal College of Physicians of London as the best screening test. The 30 item test performs well when administered in the second week after admission. It is also useful in monitoring the response to treatment. Shorter versions with 15, 10 and 4 items have been validated in primary care and continuing care. The GDS 10, administered at day 10 (when the medical state has improved) is tolerated well by inpatients. It does not require staff training. More research is needed on its utility and clinical effectiveness (Shah et al. 1997). In the four-item version, the patient is asked:

- are you basically satisfied with life?
- do you feel that your life is empty?
- are you afraid that something bad is going to happen to you?
- do you feel happy most of the time?

For the **GDS-30**, 0–10 indicates 'not depressed', 11–20 indicates 'mild depression' and 21–30 indicates 'severe depression'; for **GDS-15** a score of 5 or 6 indicates depression; for **GDS-4** a score or 1 or 2 indicates depression.

The management of depression in physically ill older people

There are few studies on the effectiveness of drugs and other therapies for depressed old people who have physical illnesses. Such studies are inherently difficult. Trials have had arbitrary age cut-offs, so there are few data on people over 80. People included in trials usually bear little relationship to the patients that physicians see in their wards and clinics.

As the evidence base for our treatment is meagre, guidelines are partly based on extrapolations of studies on younger, fitter subjects and individual clinical judgement.

General treatment

If the patients are nursed on a ward where the staff are highly motivated, skilled and caring, they are likely to feel better. Pain control, symptom relief, careful explanations, involvement in a goal-setting and decision-making will all help to improve patient well-being. Flexibility about diets, domestic pets and visiting times will reflect an imaginative approach to patient care. Being told that the aim is to improve symptoms, function and well-being, so that they can return home, will usually lift patients' spirits.

Specific treatment

A MORI poll of 2000 people found that only 16% favoured drug therapy for depression (Pitt 1997). Over three-quarters believed that these drugs were addictive. It is therefore wise to ask the depressed patient if he or she would be agreeable to a course of antidepressants before embarking on this therapy.

In cases of mild depression, active treatment is no better than placebo. In more severe depression, the first step will usually be to choose between a tricyclic antidepressant (TCA), a selective serotonin re-uptake inhibitor (SSRI), or one of the newer agents.

TCAs are more effective than placebo. One of these drugs, dothiepin, is the only agent which has been shown successfully to reduce the risk of relapses.

The TCAs are cheap but have unwelcome side-effects (falls, accidents and car-diovascular effects) which limit their use in elderly patients. They should be avoided in those with heart failure or cardiac rhythm disturbances. They should not be given to patients with suicidal ideation, as they are dangerous when taken in overdose. Of the newer TCAs, Nortriptyline seems to be well tolerated and Lofepramine has fewer anticholinergic effects. Unfortunately, the TCAs are often given in subtherapeutic doses.

SSRIs are no more effective than TCAs but are much more expensive. They have fewer *serious* side-effects, though diarrhoea and vomiting can be trou-blesome. The trials of these drugs have been carefully reviewed by Katona (1997). These drugs are generally well tolerated but there are few data on long term use. Unlike dothiepin, none of these drugs appears to prevent relapse of depression (see Chapter 4 for further details).

There are even fewer studies of more recently introduced drugs such as Venlafaxine (**NARI** – noradrenaline and serotonin re-uptake inhibitors) and Moclobemide (**RIMA** – reversible inhibitor of mono amine oxidase-A).

Whichever drug is used, patients should be warned that it may be some weeks before they notice any benefits (though some patients seem better soon after starting treatment and some of the newer drugs may have a more rapid onset of action). The medication should continue for at least 6 months and then be gradually withdrawn.

How effective are antidepressant drugs?

The most recent meta-analysis by the Cochrane Library (Gill and Hatcher 1999) reports on 18 randomized controlled trials of antidepressant versus placebo or no therapy. These studies were of adults who also had a physical illness: they did not select out trials on older people. The conclusion is that patients on anti-depressants are significantly more likely to improve than those on placebo or on no treatment. The drop-out rate was small: for 10 patients on active treat-ment, one would discontinue therapy. The drop-out rate appeared higher in TCAs than SSRIs though there was a trend for TCAs to be more effective.

The presence of physical illness does not limit the effectiveness of antide-pressant drugs (Evans et al. 1997). Though antidepressants are effective, we must be aware of their limitations including:

- In patients with mild depression, active treatment is no better than placebo.
- Some patients (especially those with severe depression) do not respond to them.
- Different patients need different doses of TCAs to effect a response (Paykel 1995).
- Some are very sensitive to these drugs, others need high doses to achieve an effect.
- Many patients discontinue their medication – they may not be aware that they should continue them for months; they may fear habituation; they may find the side-effects unacceptable.

- The relapse rate is high but can be successfully treated by a different drug in many cases.
- About a quarter of depressed older patients continue to be ill with depression despite active treatment (OADIG 1993).

When to refer to an old age psychiatrist

Most depressed older people with physical illness can be treated satisfactorily by their physician. However, there are circumstances when specialist help should be sought. These situations include:

- Depressed patients who *refuse to eat or drink*, are becoming very *retarded* or who are a *suicidal risk*. These should be considered for ECT. Though the general view is that this treatment is barbaric, it has been shown to be effective and safe. It is more efficacious than sham ECT. It does not damage the brain. If brief unilateral pulses are given, memory impairment is minimal. It can be life-saving. ECT must be considered carefully in patients who have had a recent myocardial infarction or stroke. Pacemakers are not a barrier to having ECT, nor is the use of anticoagulants (Wilkinson 1997).
- Those who remain depressed despite TCA or SSRI therapy.
- Depressed patients with delusions or hallucinations.
- Those who relapse.
- Those in whom there are diagnostic doubts.
- Those who are very agitated or who have other behavioural problems.

Where do we go from here?

The priority is to *apply* present knowledge. We now have tools which aid the recognition of depression and cheap, effective and readily available treatments that improve the life of many ill older people. We need more and better clinical trials of antidepressants in old age. These trials should:

- Consider the patient's viewpoint as well as the assessor's observations.
- Include quality of life scales and measures of activities of daily living.
- Attempt to ascertain which depressed patients respond to what types of treatment. Are there markers to identify those who are likely to be helped by drugs, psychological help or other measures?

We also need to know whom to target for cognitive behaviour therapy. Here the emphasis is on changing dysfunctional thoughts and attitudes and replacing them with more positive responses. The therapist gives the patient a series of graded assignments which can produce a sense of achievement. Cognitive therapy is more effective than placebo or no therapy and the outcomes in older people are equivalent to those in younger ones (Koder *et al*. 1996). However, we do not know which individuals are most suited to this approach.

The key to successful identification and treatment of depression in ill old people is education of medical, nursing and rehabilitation staff. Liaison psychiatric teams may have a role here but more work is needed to determine their effectiveness.

Key Points

- Depression is the commonest psychiatric problem affecting physically ill older people.
- Depression in older people may present with physical symptoms, agitation, anger, sleepiness, or poor concordance with medication.
- The diagnosis of depression is frequently overlooked and often not recorded in medical case-notes.
- Older medically ill patients have a greater mortality, morbidity and length of hospital stay. Their rehabilitation is more difficult.
- Drug treatment of depression is effective: TCAs are at least as effective as SSRIs, are much cheaper but there are more contraindications to their use in older people.
- SSRIs are helpful but have not been shown to prevent relapses. In general, treatment should continue for 6 months – longer after a relapse.
- Cognitive therapy is also more effective than placebo or no treatment but we do not know which patients are most likely to respond.
- ECT can be life saving in severely depressed patients and is generally safe.
- Optimum treatment may not occur because of suboptimal dosage, short duration of therapy, poor patient concordance or side-effects.
- In many cases, treatment of depression effects recovery. In others, recovery may be incomplete or depression may recur. Sometimes depression persists despite therapy.

References

Bowler, C., Boyle, A., Branford, M. and Cooper, S.A. (1994) Detection of psychiatric disorders in medical in-patients. *Age and Ageing*, **23**, 307–311.

Burell, P. W., Hall, W.D., Stampfer, H.G. and Emmerson, J.P. (1991) The prognosis of depression in old age. *British Journal of Psychology*, **158**, 64–71.

Davies, K.N., Burn, W.K., McKenzie, F.R., Brothwell, J.A. and Wattis, J.P. (1993) Evaluation of the Hospital Anxiety and Depression Scale as a screening instrument in geriatric medical patients. *International Journal of Geriatric Psychiatry*, **8**, 165–169.

Devinsky, O. (1992) Depression often complicates organic disease. In *Behavioural Neurology, 100 Maxims*, pp. 351–356. Edward Arnold, London.

Dinan, T.G. (1999) The physical consequences of depressive illness. *British Medical Journal*, **318**, 826.

Evans, M., Hammond, M., Wilson, K., Lye, M. and Copeland, J. (1997) Placebo-controlled treatment trial of depression in elderly physically ill depression in elderly physically ill patients. *International Journal Geriatric Psychiatry*, **12**, 817–824.

Gill, D. and Hatcher, S. (1999) Antidepressant drugs in depressed patients who also have a physical illness (Cochrane Review) In: The Cochrane Library, Issue 3 Oxford: Update Software.

Hammond, M.T., Evans, M.E. and Lye, M. (1993) Depression in medical wards. *International Journal Geriatric Psychiatry*, **8**, 957–957.

House, A. and Ebrahim, S. (1996) Psychological aspects of physical disease. In *Psychiatry in the Elderly*, edited by R. Jacoby and C. Oppenheimer, pp. 437–460. Oxford University Press, Oxford.

Irwin, M., Artin, K.H. and Oxman, M.N. (1999) Screening for depression in the older adult. Criterion validity of the 10–item center for Epidemiological Studies Depression Scale (CES-D). *Archives of Internal Medicine*, **159**, 1701–1704.

Katona, C.L.E. (1997) New antidepressants in the elderly. In *Advances in Old Age Psychiatry: Chromosomes to Community Care*, edited by C. Holmes and R. Howard, pp. 143–160. Wrightson Biomedical Publishing, Petersfield, UK.

Koder, D.-A., Brodaty, H. and Anstey, K.J. (1996) Cognitive therapy for depression in the elderly. *International Journal Geriatric Psychiatry*, **11**, 97–107.

Maguire, P. and Howell, A. (1995) Improving the psychological care of cancer patients In *Psychiatric Aspects of Physical Illness*, edited by A. House, R. Mayou and C. Mallinson, pp. 41–54. Royal College of Physicians and Royal College of Psychiatrists, London.

Mulley, G.P. and House, A. (1995) Stroke. In *Psychiatric Aspects of Physical Illness*, edited by A. House, R. Mayou and C. Mallinson, pp. 31–40. Royal College of Physicians and Royal College of Psychiatrists, London.

Old Age Depression Interest Group (1993) How long should the elderly take antidepressants? A double-blind placebo – controlled study of continuation/prophylaxis therapy with dothiepin. *British Journal Psychiatry*, **162**, 175–182.

Paykel, E.S. (1995) The place of psychoptic drug therapy. In *Psychiatric Aspects of Physical Disease*, edited by A. House, R. Mayou and C. Mallinson, pp. 69–80. Royal College of Physicians and Royal College of Psychiatrists, London.

Pitt, B. (1997) Defeating depression in old age. In *Advances in Old Age Psychiatry: Chromosomes to Community Care*, edited by C. Holmes and R. Howard, pp. 137–142. Wrightson Biomedical Publishing, Petersfield, UK.

Shah, A., Herbert, R., Lewis, S., Mahendran, R., Platt, J. and Bhattacharyya, B. (1997) Screening for depression among acutely ill geriatric patients with a short geriatric depression scale. *Age and Ageing*, **26**, 217–221.

Wilkinson, D. (1997) ECT in the elderly. In *Advances in Old Age Psychiatry: Chromosomes to Community Care*, edited by C. Holes and R. Howard, pp. 161–171.Wrightson Biomedical Publishing Ltd, Petersfield, UK.

Yohannes, A.M., Roomi, J., Baldwin, R.C., Connolly, M.J. (1998) Depression in elderly outpatients with disabling chronic obstructive pulmonary disease. *Age and Ageing*, **27**, 155–160.

The role of the clinical psychologist in the assessment, diagnosis and management of depression in older people

Carol Martin

Introduction

One of the questions any clinical psychologist gets used to is 'what is the difference between a clinical psychologist and a psychiatrist?'. Each of us develops our own typical stock response. It often goes along the lines of 'A psychiatrist is concerned with treating mental illness, while a clinical psychologist uses what we know about people to help those who are finding it difficult to cope with the problems in their lives'. The key differences between the two approaches are based in those aspects of a person's difficulties to which each attends and the theories each uses to make sense of the difficulties the sufferer describes. However, it is more complicated even than that; clinical psychologists come from an academic discipline that contains a number of theoretical frameworks. These range from an interest in how the 'hard wiring' of the brain affects behaviour; through the relationship between environment and behaviour; attitudes and beliefs held by individuals about themselves, their relationships and their actions; to the unexamined fantasies and assumptions which influence the way in which people live their life. These all offer information that is potentially useful for a clinician faced with a patient in difficulty. Some of these will clearly have more relevance for depression in late life than others, and this chapter will only cover a small proportion of the theory and research available. For those interested in pursuing these areas in more depth, including outcome research, two recent publications offer more comprehensive reviews (Edelstein 1998, Woods and Roth 1996).

The role of the clinical psychologist has developed dramatically over the last 20 years. Then, clinical psychology was a small profession in the UK and only a few chose to work with older people. Since then, there has been an increase in the size of the profession and the range of activities carried out by its members. Post-graduate training has been extended from 2 to 3 years to reflect this increase, resulting in a 6–year basic training. Experience with older people is a core component in every clinical psychologist's training. Typically, a recently qualified clinical psychologist has gained a doctorate that equips them with a range of skills in research and clinical work. After qualifying, he or she may specialize in an area defined by either specific activities or by clinical population. For example, within a large urban department there may be several clinical psychologists working with older people, each one having different strengths. These might include neuropsychological assessment, behavioural work, family therapy skills, experience of audit and other applied research skills, or training in particular therapeutic approaches.

Included in this chapter are clinical examples used to illustrate work typical of that done by clinical psychologists in Britain. All the case histories are either fictional or composites created from a number of cases. A number of assessment tools in common use are included, but the chapter does not offer an exhaustive list. Therapeutic approaches commonly used by clinical psychologists when working with individual clients are discussed, and other clinical interventions are mentioned, but again, this is not a list of what every clinical psychologist can or might do. Because the number of clinical psychologists who work with older people is small, the chapter contents cannot be taken as a guide to what is available in any particular service. Many areas of the country still have a service for older people of one whole time equivalent or less from clinical psychology. This tends to happen both as a result of funding priorities and through the recruitment difficulties common to Cinderella services.

The chapter will focus primarily on what is common to Britain but will at times make use of material from outside the UK, especially from the USA. However, because there are differences both in culture and in health provision, it cannot always be assumed that knowledge from the USA will be transferable. For example, when Reality Orientation was first developed in the USA, formal sessions were carried out in a classroom format. This did not work well for British groups, whose sessions tended to run better in an informal small group, or tea party, format (Holden and Woods 1986).

Over the years, there has been much debate over the nature of depression as a condition. This ranges from the medical understanding of depression as an illness, through to the view that depression is a normal biological and emotional response to circumstances. This debate will not be tackled in detail within this chapter, but the reader will need to bear in mind that many psychological and psychotherapeutic approaches are based on the premise that depression is not best, or is not only to be, understood as an illness. For example, the development of systemic and narrative theories has led to new therapeutic approaches, some of which are being taken up within services for older people; these theories imply that depression can be seen as a response to psychological and social conditions. Therapy then aims to understand or change these, whether through working with families or the depressed person. Some therapists are reluctant to work with people who are undergoing other treatments for depression, such as ECT, especially if the two types of treatment have different aims. For example, therapies that aim at the recognition of feelings and thoughts or the resolution of conflict may be undermined by concurrent treatments that aim to reduce feelings of distress or anxiety directly. However, there are many instances where multiple approaches are helpful, e.g. medication and cognitive therapy combined.

Assessment and diagnosis

Medical diagnoses and methods of assessment have been discussed in Chapters 1and 2. When an individual is referred to a clinical psychologist, he or she will be assessed again. This assessment will vary depending on the:

- source of the referral;
- previous and current contact with services; and
- skills and perspective of the particular psychologist.

Referrals tend to have their origins in one of two types of service. The first type comes through psychiatric services, community mental health teams or other specialist health service staff. The second type is the primary care referral, made usually by a general practitioner, but sometimes by staff, such as a district nurse, or by someone outside the NHS, e.g. from social service or voluntary organizations. It is quite likely that this will lead to some differences in the assessment procedure. For example, in the first type of referral, there will already be a psychiatric diagnosis, the person may already be taking and responding to medication, and there may be other staff from the service already involved. On the other hand, when someone's first contact with mental health services is with a clinical psychologist, it is likely that the clinician will be considering the psychiatric aspects of depression while assessing the psychological conditions. If there are significant psychiatric concerns, a request may be made for additional input from psychiatry or from the team.

A psychological assessment may include a number of areas (Table 8.1). It is almost never carried out in a mechanistic way; assessment needs to take into account the complexity and individuality of human experience. A full assessment may take several sessions, especially if formal assessment measures are used, or if a trial of therapy is included in the assessment period. For a depressed person, an assessment of mood will be included, often using a standard measure. The information gained within the assessment should allow the clinician to build a model of the relationship between the patient's distress and symptoms and other relevant aspects of an individual's situation. This is a *formulation*, the psychologist's equivalent of diagnosis. Unlike a diagnosis, it is usually expressed in dynamic terms, and often includes a description of the processes that exacerbate or maintain distress or symptomatology. A formulation will vary depending on:

- the presentation of the patient;
- other evidence available to the clinician; and
- the theoretical framework used by the clinician.

For example, a clinician using a behavioural framework would be concerned to elicit details of the triggers for and consequences of the behaviours in question. The formulation has a role in enabling therapist and client to agree goals and strategies for change and is itself constantly being updated and modified in the light of experience.

Table 8.1. Areas for assessment.

Mood and emotions	e.g. Hopelessness, despair, anger, lability of emotion.
Cognitive functioning	e.g. Memory. Planning and abstraction.
Thoughts and beliefs	e.g. Beliefs about self, others and the future. Attributional style.
Behaviour	e.g. Risky behaviour, self harm. Activity levels.
Past history	e.g. Past emotional disturbance. Relationship and work life.
Interpersonal style	e.g. Presence and quality of marital relationship, friendships. Attachment style.
Current circumstances	e.g. Ill health and consequent limitations. Family, marital and social support. Areas of anxiety, e.g. finances.
Life events	e.g. Retirement, bereavement, deprivation, loss, change in living circumstances, trauma.
Resources	Strengths and needs.
Readiness for therapy	e.g. curiosity about self and psychology, willingness to give something a try.

Use of questionnaires

Many of the assessments of mood state have been devised for younger adult populations, but there are now several that have been standardized for use with older people. Probably, the questionnaires most commonly used by clinical psychologists in the UK are the:

- Beck Depression Inventory (BDI);
- Geriatric Depression Scale (GDS); and
- Hospital Anxiety and Depression Scale (HADS).

The **BDI** and other related scales are often selected because of their basis in cognitive models of depression. This means that the questionnaire can sometimes elicit responses that may be useful to explore further in therapy. It has been validated for use with older people (Gallagher *et al.* 1982). The **GDS** (Yesavage *et al.* 1983) is a yes/no self-report scale, simpler than the BDI and increasingly used, especially now that shorter forms are being developed. The **HADS** has several advantages. It is short, and it includes items for rating anxiety as well as depression. Other professions also commonly use it, so that the results are easily communicated. Descriptions of these and other scales for mood and well-being are described in Woods (1999).

The role of neuropsychological testing in depression of older people; depression or dementia – or both?

One of the most common reasons for an older person to be referred to a clinical psychologist is so that the reasons for a reduced capacity to function in everyday life can be clarified. Often the question is framed as 'Is this person suffering from dementia or depression?'. This often necessitates one or more periods of neuropsychological assessment. An initial conversation will give the psychologist an idea of how well the person is likely to be able to manage when being assessed; the initial choice of test may be decided when the person is first seen. The choice of tests is dependent also on the function of the testing. For example, the referral may involve diagnostic purposes only; in this case, it is likely that a relatively standard battery of tests that ascertain how well the person is doing compared to others of their age and pre-morbid ability will be sufficient. However, if the testing aims to specify intact abilities, particular areas of difficulty or patterns of deficit, or if the intention is to use the assessment in order to design programmes which help the person adapt and cope in spite of their deficits, a different range of tests may be useful. In practice, those people referred to clinical psychology for assistance with diagnosis often present a complex or ill-defined picture and the results of testing can be equivocal. It is also fairly common for someone to be suffering from both conditions. Woods (1999) discusses findings that suggest that there is a group of individuals with depression who also show cognitive changes on testing which are not consistent with dementia. Their scores fall between those achieved by those with either 'depression only' or 'dementia only'. In such circumstances, it is often better for any treatment for depression to be pursued first. Detailed testing can then be carried out at a point where a more accurate picture of the type and degree of organic impairment is possible. Assessments repeated over time may also be helpful. Woods (1999) and Crawford *et al.* (1998) offer comprehensive and up-to-date descriptions of the benefits and limitations of neuropsychological testing and of the strengths of the tests available for use with an older population. Both chapters include more detailed discussion of the issues involved in the differentiation of organic from functional conditions.

Commonly used cognitive screening tests

For a quickly administered and acceptable screening test when the cognitive status of a depressed person is in doubt, the **Middlesex Elderly Assessment of Mental State (MEAMS)** (Golding 1989) is a possible choice. There are other screening tests for cognitive functioning, such as the **Clifton Assessment Procedure for the Elderly (CAPE)** (Pattie and Gilleard 1979) or **the Mini-Mental State Examination (MMSE)** (Folstein *et al.* 1975), some of which are also used by other professions.

The **Health Questionnaire, SF-36**, which has often been used in research populations, has a short section on mental health. This correlates well with other scales and is a possible choice where health is an issue. However, questionnaires are best viewed as a supplementary form of information on the client's state. They are certainly insufficient as the sole basis for a psychological formulation without the additional information gained through interviews and observations. See Woods (1999) for references concerning these and other tests and Case History 8.1 for an example of their use in clinical practice.

The role of the clinical psychologist in the management of depression

The interventions offered by clinical psychologists to the management of depression in older people include both:

- direct client work; and
- indirect work.

Direct client work may consist of individual and group work. One or more of a number of therapeutic frameworks may inform clinical work with depressed older people. Indirect work may also take a number of forms. These include supervision of the work of others; training; consultation; work with staff and carers on the environment; and research. A number of areas of psychology have relevance for these endeavours.

Case History 8.1

Mrs Green was referred for neuropsychological assessment following an admission to hospital. A CPN had been asked to see her at home, where he found her depressed and clearly not coping. She had stopped consistent self-care and seemed withdrawn and slow. This continued while on the ward, where she was withdrawn, slow and reluctant to engage in any activity. The staff were puzzled by her behaviour. She was treated with antidepressant medication. After several weeks, there was a slight improvement, so that Mrs Green was a little more able to look after herself, but not consistently. Moreover, she was still low in mood and reluctant to talk with staff. The initial screen for cognitive functioning used by the junior doctor had given a score well below normal, but he had found it difficult to be sure that this was an accurate picture of Mrs Green's level of functioning, particularly as Mrs Green was reluctant to attempt many items. It was felt that a more complete assessment might cast light on her condition, before considering further treatments for depression. The psychologist saw Mrs Green initially to try to form a picture of relevant history. She also wanted to explain the need for testing and what it might involve, given that it can be a long procedure and that the active co-operation of the patient is necessary throughout. While Mrs Green attempted to talk of the details of her history, the psychologist found herself interested in the details of Mrs Green's way of telling her story as much as the content. Mrs Green spoke very slowly. In fact, she did everything slowly. Her mood seemed flat. She complained of memory loss. When asked for examples, she talked of difficulties when carrying out everyday tasks, such as returning to turn off the taps when running a bath, or letting pans boil dry. She was anxious about coping at home and feared that she might be sent to live in an institution. When the psychologist reassured her that the testing was not intended to show her incompetence, and might even help staff to develop possible strategies for coping at home, she relaxed and was keen to continue. When asked about her mood, she said that she thought she was not as she had been before she became depressed, but felt she was much better than she had been at the time of admission. A depression scale confirmed this. On testing, she showed relatively little memory loss. She did have some difficulty with more complex reading, writing and arithmetic. There were no indications of problems with comprehension or expression, whether of visual or verbal material. She did perform poorly on a test requiring the capacity to think in abstract terms. The psychologist concluded that Mrs Green did not show on testing a pattern typical of Alzheimer's disease but she did feel concerned that Mrs Green was performing less well than she might have expected on some tests. The pattern seemed more consistent with a sub-cortical state, and she discussed this with the medical staff. She involved the team's Occupational Therapist and they continued to see Mrs Green, discussing her difficulties with her and developing ways of helping her to adapt more successfully to her home environment. This included the use of memory aids and prompts, some developed following home visits. Mrs Green improved relatively rapidly, although she remained slow and her cognitive functioning did not change dramatically. When she was discharged, she began to cope successfully at home. Some time later, Mrs Green began to demonstrate more clearly the symptoms of Parkinson's disease. However, she continued to live at home for several years.

Clinical work with individuals

Most therapeutic work currently done by clinical psychologists with depressed older people can be classed as belonging to one of two main groupings:

- cognitive–behavioural; and
- psychodynamic–interpersonal.

Woods and Roth (1996) have carried out a major review of the evidence for the outcome of psychotherapy with older people. They report on a number of studies researching the prevalence and prognosis of depression in old age, and conclude from the evidence that prevalence rates for depression are similar in older people to those found in younger people. The natural history of depression in older people may be less favourable, there being a substantial number whose depression does not recover with the standard (medical) treatments, and with relapse being a major issue (Woods and Roth 1996, p. 322). They note that older people seem less likely to receive psychological treatment. The research that has been done seems to them to suggest that older people can make use of the psychological approaches used with younger populations, although progress may be slower. They conclude that the results from the few available controlled trials suggest that brief psychodynamic psychotherapy, cognitive therapy and behaviour therapy appear to be equally effective for treating depression in older people. In this instance, brief therapy typically involves agreeing on a therapeutic focus and a contract of up to 20 sessions.

It is worth bearing in mind that a number of factors may militate against referral for psychological therapy. The existence of waiting lists may reduce referral rates. Many of those who are referred for therapy are among those who fail to respond to standard treatments. They may therefore need longer treatments, and clinicians who are experienced in work with complex or resistant conditions. Even so, the rates for improvement may not be high with this group. Further, older people are perhaps less likely to welcome a psychological approach to their difficulties. There may be a number of reasons for this, ranging from the idea that emotional and personal matters should not be discussed with others, to the wish to avoid dependence on others or anxiety about being seen by others as vulnerable or foolish. Therapy needs to be seen by patient and referrer as an appropriate response to the problem. Indeed, the early stages of therapy usually involve finding a shared view of the problem. This may be linked to the finding, cited by Woods and Roth, that 'patient commitment' to therapy is a significant factor in predicting outcome of treatment in depressed older people (Marmar et al. 1989). In particular, the propensity for depressive symptomatology to be seen as physical by older people and others may make a psychological formulation seem inappropriate or disrespectful unless it is carefully constructed (see Case History 8.2).

Case History 8.2

Mrs Jones was referred with a long history of complaints of pain and symptoms attributed by her doctors to tension. She also felt fatigue and constipation. Initially, she was resistant to the idea that a psychological approach would be helpful with what seemed to her to be a series of physical symptoms. She felt rejected and let down by her doctors for referring her to a psychologist because she felt this meant that they disbelieved her and could not help her. She felt sure that, as her symptoms felt physical, there must be a medical solution for them. The psychologist was faced with the dilemma that Mrs Jones would not accept any formulation that seemed to discount the physical nature of her symptoms, while one that accepted her point of view left little room for intervention. He decided to take a neutral stance towards the cause of the symptoms, suggesting that any monitoring of the symptoms would be useful in order to find out whether there were triggers, but that should the symptoms be physical in origin, the information might be helpful in diagnosis. Mrs Jones agreed to keep a diary of her symptoms. As it turned out, it became clear from the diary that there were a number of environmental and emotional triggers. For example, Mrs Jones recorded that her symptoms often worsened at the end of visits and trips. This was particularly true for those symptoms most easily attributable to anxiety. The psychologist suggested she might be anxious about being left alone. Mrs Jones agreed that she became frightened of becoming ill and unable to contact help. Some of her anxieties and symptoms provoked others in a vicious cycle. Once this was noted, and the psychologist worked out with Mrs Jones the possible relationship between her symptoms and feelings of anxiety, Mrs Jones agreed to try relaxation exercises. During this period, it became clear that there were ways in which Mrs Jones behaved that reduced anxiety in the short term, but at a cost to herself. For example, she insisted that a family member accompany her when she went out. Consequently she had lost many of her old activities and friendships, and she felt unable to take up opportunities for new ones. Her mood was often low, she became easily discouraged when her symptoms started and she complained repeatedly about how awful her life had become. The psychologist asked her to try out some small behavioural changes. The first of these were chosen in order that Mrs Jones might become used to success before trying goals that were more uncertain. After a number of setbacks, Mrs Jones began to accept that she could help herself to feel better and that,she did have the necessary skills for coping with both her symptoms and for making her life more satisfying. Over a period of a year or so, she began to reorganize her social life and renew links with others.

Cognitive–behavioural and cognitive therapies

Cognitive and cognitive–behavioural approaches are probably the most commonly available therapies offered by clinical psychology services for older people. The vignette above describes part of a therapy based in the main on cognitive–behavioural principles. The approach initially developed by Aaron Beck is probably the most well known. Increasingly, the practice of cognitive therapy is becoming more sophisticated, and there are now specialist trainings, which provide therapists with a thorough grounding in the theory and practice of cognitive therapy. However, because the principles seem simple, and have an appeal, many practitioners in mental health incorporate techniques from cognitive therapy into their repertoire. Cognitive therapy has been used successfully with people who suffer from depression without manic or psychotic disturbance (Hawton *et al.* 1989).

Basic ideas and premises

Cognitive therapists act on the assumption that the beliefs people have about the world and themselves influence their feelings and their behaviour. Given that depression is a state brought about and affected by biological, social, developmental and psychological factors, cognitions are one potential, powerful, focus for intervention. The therapist and client need to form a collaborative relationship; the rationale of cognitive therapy needs to make sense to the client. Each has an active part to play in therapy. Cognitive therapies are usually:

- short and time-limited;
- focused on current problems and the factors that maintain them;
- involve the therapist asking questions;
- encourage the client to consider their thoughts and beliefs as hypotheses that can be tested; and
- facilitate systematic experimentation.

The aim is for clients to develop the skills necessary to help themselves. Once the client learns the principles of the approach, it is assumed that the process can be continued without regular input from the therapist. Cognitive therapy sessions revolve around the identification of a focus, selection of a strategy for tackling it, discussing the implementation of the strategy, which may include the setting of homework, and monitoring the outcome. This, when it goes well, becomes a benign spiral, where problem-solving skills and constructive assumptions about the relationship between thought, behaviour and feelings are developed by the client, who may then go on to use what has been learned in the sessions for other problems as necessary.

Adaptations with older people

Older people may take longer to grasp the relevance of therapy techniques and to complete planned tasks. Sometimes external supports and health problems intervene. It is sometimes necessary to be more flexible about the frequency and duration of individual sessions and the therapy as a whole. Making sure that communication is effective is important, whether any difficulties are due to physical problems, such as deafness, or social and cultural ones, such as differences in language or background. In practice, sessions for behavioural and cognitive techniques can be spread out without too much difficulty, although it is important to make sure that a sense of continuity is maintained. Group work has been used successfully with older people (Yost *et al.* 1986). Many psychologists working with older people seem to find a contract for fortnightly sessions optimal. For many older people, there seems to be a phase in even a structured therapy when it seems that talking of wider issues and troubles is important. Sometimes a session when the client talks of other matters and the planned task takes a back seat, turns out, in retrospect, to have been very influential.

Recently, there have been attempts to discover the most useful concepts from cognitive therapy that are most useful for older people. For example, recently, there has been an interest in the ways in which people maintain pleasurable mood states and self esteem. James *et al.* (1999) suggest that the failure of previously successful mechanisms for maintaining self-esteem, which they call Worth Enhancing Belief Systems (WEBS), may be a more important factor in depression which appears later in life, than negative automatic thoughts (see Case History 8.3).

Case History 8.3

Mr Stevens was referred with depressed mood and anxiety. He had been attending the Day Hospital, but was reluctant to be discharged. He had moved into sheltered housing soon after the death of his wife several years before. During the initial interview, he complained that he did not like being alone in the flat. Indeed, a diary of his daily activities collected later, showed that he spent very little time there. The time he did spend in the flat was taken up with housework, except for cooking. He ate his meals out, with friends, at the Day Hospital, the Day Centre, or even out alone. This was in contrast to his life before his wife's death, when he had spent the majority of his time at home, watching television and pursuing a number of leisure activities. While a psychodynamic formulation might have emphasized his difficulty in tolerating being left alone with his feelings, and focused on exploring this, it was decided that Mr Stevens might more easily accept a cognitive–behavioural approach, at least initially. He was asked to keep an activity diary. He was also asked to compile a list of activities he had previously enjoyed; he then rated these in terms of how much he had enjoyed each and how practical it would be to resume each. Homework for this task involved collecting the necessary materials for a number of these, so that they were readily available in the flat. The next step was to programme into his routines a short time period each day when he would stay in the flat. The idea was that this would gradually be increased. After the first attempt, Mr Stevens came to his next session complaining that he had felt terrible and had had to go out. After discussion, he and the psychologist agreed that he would try again, but keep a record of his thoughts and feelings during the few minutes he was required to stay in alone. Although the content of the record was not very useful in itself, the ensuing discussion made more sense of his experience. Mr Stevens admitted that he felt abandoned and lonely after the death of his wife. He and the therapist identified how he felt helpless and weak when these feelings came up. The additional complication was the fact that Mr Stevens also felt angry that he was in this position. He was several years older than his wife and had expected to die before her. Mr Stevens admitted that his wife had been a nervous woman, who had hated being alone; he had therefore always stayed in with her. This meant he had neither developed friendships and activities outside the home, nor had he had previously to face his own anxieties about being alone. He had not anticipated having to face all this, and he was anxious that he would die alone. Once this was out in the open, the practical issues about living

Case History 8.3 Continued.

alone could be discussed. It was also important, however, when Mr Stevens confided that he had always felt insecure inside. Once he began to see part of his current experience as a remnant of childhood experience, like sleeping alone in the dark, it could be re-evaluated in that light. He could be satisfied by realistic appraisals of his safety. While Mr Stevens never came to like living alone, he did find himself able to spend time at home in useful and pleasant occupations, and began to invite friends to visit him. His mood lifted and he began to accept those pleasures still available to him.

Psychodynamic and interpersonal therapies

Basic ideas and premises

These therapies are offered when the problems of the patient are understood to be in terms of difficulties in relationships, difficulties adapting to current life circumstances or can be seen as internal to the individual. A core feature is the recognition that individuals facing a reality that feels intolerable will often protect themselves by distorting their understanding or their experience. Everybody has to do this at times, and some strategies are more constructive than others. Some types of strategy, or defence, are more easily tolerated and more easily reversible than others. Those seeking a general introduction to psychodynamic therapy may read Malan (1979). Therapies of this type are intended to allow a person to understand themselves and their situation better. Sometimes, as a consequence, someone may develop previously unexpressed qualities, or a new perspective on life. The role of the therapist may vary from providing an environment in which someone feels safe to talk and reflect, to offering interpretations. The more psychoanalytically informed, the more likely it is that the therapist will think about the experience of both participants in the therapeutic relationship, i.e. in terms of transference and counter-transference. Genevay and Katz (1990) have collected a number of essays on these phenomena in relation to older people. Instances of therapeutic work with older people can be found in Knight (1986, 1992). Psychotherapy with older people has some features exclusive to work with this group. The nature of the goals and the tasks facing older people differs. For example, a young widow might be expecting to develop a career and to find a new partner, while an older widow may need to adapt to living alone, finding new leisure activities and maintaining her friendships. There is likely to be a generational difference between the client and the therapist; sometimes a gap may cover several generations. This often colours the relationship between therapist and client in subtle ways, as the two try to make sense of the situation in which they find themselves. For example, an older client may think of the therapist as an adult child, or even a grandchild. This may have effects on the progress of therapy; patients may feel unwilling to talk of difficulties if they feel anxious that a younger person may not understand; or they may feel protective towards this young person, who should not have to know such painful things. Clinical psychology, like other mental health professions, is a young discipline. Many NHS staff will be up to 70 years younger than the patients they see. Gaps in understanding and experience are likely in all helping relationships, but patient and professional are part of a society that accepts a number of prejudices about age, and both staff and patients may have beliefs that affect the quality and effect of health care. Sometimes it is possible to sort out difficulties by providing information. On occasion, however, a role may develop because it has benefits for the patient's mood and reduces the anxiety of both patient and professional. When such a situation develops without being understood, the concepts of transference and counter-transference can be useful (Genevay and Katz 1990). Sometimes referrals to clinical psychology are made when other helping relationships have been impeded by such distortions and difficulties.

Knight (1986) and Orbach (1996) have written good introductions to the field of psychotherapy with older people. Even outside a formal psychotherapeutic contract, there are often benefits from a formulation that includes some of the concepts from psychodynamic psychotherapy. A psychodynamic formulation can sometimes make sense of what seems at first sight to be perverse, challenging or bizarre behaviour, for example. It may be possible then to offer ordinary care in a way that is more comfortable for carer and patient.

Adaptations for work with older people

A number of issues are common to work with older people. The elderly are usually defined as those over 65 (60 for women). This includes individuals whose ages range through a period of 35 years or more. Each age group has different experiences, and historical events sometimes combine with the cohort effect to produce generations whose experiences are quite different from those who are born earlier or later. For example, boys born in the period between 1910 and 1920 were young men at the start of World War II, and their common experience is soldiering. Therapists working with these men as they have aged commonly hear stories of war-time experiences, followed by the sequelae of such stress and the requirements to adjust back into civilian life after the war. Those born in the late 1920s and early 1930s were still children when the war started. These individuals are now entering their sixties. As a consequence, separation in childhood, due to evacuation, has become a more common issue in therapy, as it has recently in the public arena. The effects on these groups of the war has therefore led to different vulnerabilities and this requires psychologists to draw on different theoretical frameworks for making sense of this. Bowlby's (e.g. 1973) work on separation and loss in children has direct relevance for the younger group, while models for understanding the effects of trauma have face validity for work with the older group.

Psychodynamic, narrative and other interpersonal approaches can be particularly appropriate when the patient feels it necessary to talk about and reconsider earlier experience. Many such therapies are more concerned with acceptance, developing meaning and extending self-knowledge; external changes may be small. Some potential improvements may be impeded by life circumstances. However, the chance to reach some kind of resolution of their inner distress can be experienced as invaluable by some patients (see Case History 8.4).

Case History 8.4

Mrs Smith was referred to the community mental health team with depression, which had been problematic periodically throughout her adult life. This current episode had begun 4 years after the death of her husband. She made a good relationship with Sally, the CPN, who visited her at home. Mrs Smith had been timid all her life and had often given in to others to keep the peace. Mrs Smith's daughter, Jean, could not visit as regularly as Mrs Smith would like. Mrs Smith became anxious that, by confronting her daughter, she risked an argument and then losing the few visits she had. She saw her daughter as an assertive woman, like her late husband. Some strategies people use to deal with situations they find difficult are more comprehensible and more constructive than others. From the possible strategies available to her, which would both allow her to reduce her anxiety about rejection and to communicate her dissatisfaction, Mrs Smith chose to confide in the CPN. She initially said that she thought that her daughter would have visited more often, but her son-in-law had poor health and that Jean could not cope with caring for both her husband and herself. Confiding in the nurse allowed Mrs Smith to recognize and discuss her feelings of disappointment. It is possible that she might then she find ways in which to tolerate her feelings more easily. For example, she might have been able to consider ways of increasing her contact with others, so that she did not feel as lonely and as dependent on her daughter. However, it may be instead that Sally comes to take the role of a more loving daughter for Mrs Smith, one who visits regularly, listens and is understanding. This could be transference, in that it is a feeling based on Mrs Smith's wish for a daughter who will satisfy her needs, and it may well be a situation that is not understood by either Mrs Smith or Sally in this way. Most of the time it may not matter that Sally has become so important for Mrs Smith. In fact, such a relationship may be helpful to Mrs Smith's mood, and it is possible that, once feeling better, Mrs Smith may find it easier to accept her situation or rebuild her social life. Understanding more covert aspects of the relationship between the two may not then be necessary. However, let us assume that, after a while, Sally noticed that there was relatively little progress in these areas and that, furthermore, Mrs Smith periodically became more reluctant to get out of bed, withdrew from her routine and complained, about her life, her health and her family. Sally became puzzled, as she could find no reason for this. One December she visited to find Mrs Smith in bed, distressed, after a visit from her daughter. Among other complaints, Mrs Smith said that Jean had criticized her, and had told her to 'pull her socks up or she would not be welcome for Christmas'. Concerned that Mrs Smith did not improve over the next fortnight, Sally took the problem to the team meeting for discussion, worrying that Mrs Smith might become severely depressed over the holiday, perhaps needing admission to hospital. After some discussion, the psychologist, who was interested in psychodynamics, suggested the possibility that the problem times might be related to breaks. Sally considered this and remembered that the last episode like this was, in fact, just before her summer holiday. The team then realized how important Sally had become to Mrs Smith. Sally arranged to talk with the psychologist later, and then, prepared with ideas and possible comments, she returned to see Mrs Smith.

Case History 8.4 Continued.

She found an opportunity to talk with Mrs Smith about the break. The two of them considered how difficult it was for Mrs Smith, in that even when she visited Jean, she found Jean preoccupied with the care of her husband. Mrs Smith was able to talk about the shame she felt when she was angry at having to take second place, and how she berated herself for her 'ingratitude and selfishness'. She acknowledged that sometimes she retreated in protest, thinking 'why bother, if you're alone, there's no point'. She talked of how she and Jean had argued recently. It became clear to Sally that Jean was becoming the 'bad' daughter, who did not do as Mrs Smith wanted, while Mrs Smith was treating Sally as if she was the 'good' daughter. At one point, Mrs Smith said sadly that she wishes that the CPN were her daughter. This allowed Sally to discuss the nature and limits of the professional relationship with Mrs Smith. Mrs Smith agreed that although it was frustrating that she could not have a closer relationship with Sally, it was the professional nature of their relationship which meant that Mrs Smith could have their time together for talking and thinking only about her own needs. Jean, with all the other demands on her, could not manage this, and wanted to be able to confide in her mother herself. This enabled Mrs Smith to consider just how helpful her daughter was trying to be, in spite of her situation. Mrs Smith remembered how she had only recently refused to listen to Jean's troubles. They ended the session with sad feelings, but with a stronger sense of working together. Mrs Smith returned to her usual routine. Her depression lifted and she managed Christmas well. When Sally visited in the New Year, Mrs Smith told her that the visit with Jean had gone well and that Jean had appreciated her mother's support. Mrs Smith said sadly that she was not always as kind a mother as she wanted to be, but she was pleased that she was still able to '*make things a bit right*'.

Consultation

There are occasions when a clinical psychologist may be asked to add a perspective or to offer advice, rather than to see a patient individually for therapy. Sometimes this may involve neuropsychological testing, but this is not always the case. In the Case History below, the clinical psychologist felt that it would take too long and be too uncertain to work individually with the patient and that the best approach was to support the ward staff most closely involved with the patient. This can be an extremely effective way of using limited resources (see Case History 8.5).

Other approaches to patient care

Clinical psychologists are often concerned to promote a psychological perspective throughout the NHS service in which they work. This can involve them in activities other than individual assessments or therapies. Such activities include the *development and evaluation of new therapeutic approaches*. The current interest in developing psychological therapies for people with dementia is one example. This was first done systematically in the late 1970s,

Case History 8.5

The nurses involved with Mrs Brown's care were concerned about the lack of progress they were seeing in her condition. She had been on the ward for some time, very depressed, and no treatment offered thus far seemed to bring about any sustained improvement. They asked the psychologist to help them, and when she visited the ward, she found a depressed, partially immobile woman, who averted her gaze and refused to talk with her. Mrs Brown had been admitted following discharge home from hospital following a stroke. She had failed to cope in her own home, but would not consider alternative accommodation. Ward staff reported that her state varied. At times, she seemed to improve, only to relapse again. Only one of the staff, a recently qualified nurse called Karen, felt she had been able to make a positive relationship with Mrs Brown. She was keen to work with Mrs Brown, who often made eye contact with her and was sometimes willing to talk to her. Karen felt uncertain about listening; although she had done some counselling she felt concerned that she might not know how to respond therapeutically to Mrs Brown at times. It was agreed that she and the other staff involved with Mrs Brown's care would meet with the psychologist weekly for 3 weeks to discuss ways in which their care might be tailored to meet Mrs Brown's needs and condition. After the first of these meetings, the group began to develop an understanding of the circumstances to which Mrs Brown responded best. They began to work more consistently and systematically to promote these conditions whenever possible. In the second meeting, they recognized a cycle in which Mrs Brown began to improve, but became discouraged and depressed again as she began to attempt activities which she would have found easy before her stroke. By the third meeting, Mrs Brown was beginning to relate to other staff and had started to become involved in self-care and ward activities more consistently. The group then felt that it was possible to consider other approaches. Karen still had the closest relationship with Mrs Brown and she was now confident about seeing Mrs Brown for counselling, while meeting the psychologist regularly to discuss her work. Karen was initially concerned that Mrs Brown would become very upset when she realized she would not be able to cope at home again. However, after several sessions, Mrs Brown announced that she would like to consider residential care and accepted help so that she could visit possible Homes and choose one that would suit her needs. Karen continued to see Mrs Brown while she was on the ward, and then arranged to visit her twice within the Home in order to give Mrs Brown some continuity and a chance to talk over the move.

when Reality Orientation (RO) was introduced from the USA, where it had been developed to assist people with memory problems to remember the basic details of their environment. In the UK, this was adapted for wards. RO had two strands, formal sessions and a general approach, called by some '24 hour RO'. The latter was conducted by staff on the wards, while formal sessions were run by ward staff and others (Holden and Woods 1986). One effect of such groups for the members was an increase in engagement and socialization. It was clear that, even though some inpatients may not have been clinically depressed, they were clearly not functioning at their optimum level. These patients could be assumed to be feeling demoralized. Since then, there have been a number of attempts to develop ward-based regimes or therapy approaches that aim to increase the level of activity or quality of life of inpatients or day-patients. Life review, reminiscence, validation and resolution therapy all aim to enable the older person with dementia cope better with some aspect of their experience that may otherwise lead to or maintain depressed mood (Woods 1999). Moreover, there is often a role for treatment of people who attend memory clinics and their carers, who may be depressed.

Promising research

Clinical psychology draws on academic psychology as well as the applied research generated within the discipline. Attachment theory and developmental psychology are commonly used as frameworks for making sense of clinical work. Recent developments from the social sciences have also contributed to our knowledge of ageing (Pratt and Norris 1994). Academics within psychology have been using qualitative techniques to enhance our understanding of ageing. One example of research with possible implications for understanding the appearance and form of depression in older people is that of Carol Sherrard (1998), who has begun to analyse the strategies used by older people in relation to their well-being. Narrative research has also influenced the form of therapies in recent years (for example, Coleman *et al.* 1998) and has relevance for therapies such as life review (Viney 1993).

Key points

- The type of service offered in any one area will vary, dependent on the number, experience and training of the available clinical psychology staff and the skills of the other professionals with whom they work.

Clinical psychologists may:

- assist in the provision of specialized therapies, such as cognitive therapy groups, either independently or with staff from other professions;
- provide an opportunity for staff who facilitate groups to discuss the process and difficulties;
- supervise the work of those who carry out individual counselling, sometimes enabling someone who may have a good relationship with a patient to use a model of work in which they have relatively little training or direct experience;
- assist those who work with patients whose situation is complex, to think through the possibilities for therapeutic input, and avoid some of the potential difficulties, e.g. reflective practice groups;
- facilitate groups in which staff are able to discuss issues in their clinical work or in their environments, e.g. staff support groups;
- carry out research in order to understand patients' conditions better, e.g. by sampling from patient populations, or by surveying need within the population as a whole – they may assess the outcome of aspects of treat-

ment, e.g. by measuring patients' symptomatology or other aspects of their experience before and after a treatment, or by surveying patients to ascertain the strengths and shortcomings of the service they receive;

- contribute to the process of developing and monitoring policies and standards within the service;
- assist staff and carers to develop environments in which the self esteem of older people is not undermined;
- give advice on patients in whom there are psychological factors implicated in the treatment of physical health problems, e.g. non-compliance.

- Over the last 20 years, the profession has begun to develop a number of roles and activities that are of benefit to those depressed older people who can take advantage of a psychological approach.
- Clinical psychologists undertake other activities that may affect the environments in which depressed older people find themselves and may improve the psychological aspects of the care offered to them. Sometimes the benefits from therapy may not include symptom reduction, but many patients value the opportunity to examine the emotional and psychological aspects of their condition.
- In spite of limited numbers, the roles for clinical psychologists working with older people continue to develop, and there are some isolated but promising projects within the community and in health settings. Possible areas for development include a role in primary care, health promotion and prevention of depression. Hopefully the profession will continue to make its contribution, increasing the possibility that older people will be able to live a more contented old age.

References

Bowlby, J. (1973) Separation: anxiety and anger. Vol. 2 of *Attachment and Loss*. Hogarth Press, London. Penguin, Harmondsworth (1975).

Coleman, P. G., Ivani-Chalian, C. and Robinson, M. (1998) The story continues: persistence of life themes in old age. *Ageing and Society*, **18**, 389–420.

Crawford, J.R., Venneri, A. and O'Carroll, R.E. (1998) Neuropsychological assessment of the elderly. In *Clinical Geropsychology*. Volume 7 in *Comprehensive Clinical Psychology*, edited by B. Edelstein. Pergamon, Oxford.

Edelstein, B. (1998) (ed.) Clinical Geropsychology. Volume 7 in *Comprehensive Clinical Psychology*. Series edited by A.S. Bellack and M. Hersen. Pergamon, Oxford.

Erikson, E. (1968) *Identity: Youth and Crisis*. Norton, New York.

Folstein, M.F., Folstein, S.E. and McHugh, P. R. (1975) 'Mini-Mental State': a practical method for grading the cognitive state of patients for the clinician. *Journal of Psychiatric Research*, **12**, 189–198.

Gallagher, D., Nies, G. and Thompson, L.W. (1982) Reliability of the Beck depression inventory with older adults. *Journal of Consulting and Clinical Psychology*, **50**, 152–153.

Genevay, B. and Katz, R.S. (1990) (eds) *Counter-transference and Older Clients*. Sage, London.

Golding, E. (1989) *Middlesex Elderly Assessment of Mental State*. Thames Valley Test Company, Titchfield.

Hawton, K., Salkovskis, P. M., Kirk, J. and Clark, D.M. (1989) *Cognitive Behaviour Therapy for Psychiatric Problems: A Practical Guide*. Oxford University Press, Oxford.

Holden, U.P. and Woods, R.T. (1986) *Reality Orientation*. 2nd edn., Churchill Livingstone, London.

James, I.A., Kendell, K. and Reichelt, F.K. (1999) Conceptualizations of depression in older people: the interaction of positive and negative beliefs. *Behavioural and Cognitive Psychotherapy*, **27**, 285–290.

Kenn, C., Wood, H., Kucyj, M., Wattis, J.P. and Cunane, J. (1987) Validation of the Hospital Anxiety and Depression Scale (HADS) in an elderly psychiatric population. *International Journal of Geriatric Psychiatry*, **2**, 189–193.

Knight, B. (1986) *Psychotherapy with Older Adults*. Sage, London.

Knight, B. G. (1992) *Older Adults In Psychotherapy: Case Histories*. Sage, London.

Malan, D. H. (1979) *Individual Psychotherapy and the Science of Psychodynamics*. Butterworths, London.

Marmar, C.R., Gaston, L., Gallagher, D. and Thompson, L.W. (1989) Alliance and outcome in late-life depression. *Journal of Nervous and Mental Disease*, **177**, 464–472.

Orbach, A. (1996) *Not Too Late: Psychotherapy and Ageing*. Jessica Kingsley, London.

Pattie, A. and Gilleard, C.J. (1979) *Manual for the Clifton assessment Procedures for the Elderly*. Hodder and Stoughton Educational, Sevenoaks.

Pratt, M.W. and Norris, J.E. (1994) *The Social Psychology of Ageing*, Blackwell.

Sherrard, C. A. (1998) Strategies for well-being in later life: a qualitative analysis. *British Journal of Medical Psychology*, **71**, 253–263.

Viney, L. L. (1993) *Life Stories: Personal Construct Therapy With The Elderly*. Wiley, Chichester.

Woods, R.T. and Roth, A. (1996) Effectiveness of psychological interventions with older people. In *What Works for Whom? A Critical Review of Psychotherapy Research*, edited by A. Roth and P. Fonagy, 321-340. Guilford Press, London.

Woods, R.T. (1999) Psychological assessment of older people. In *Psychological Problems of Ageing: Assessment, Treatment and Care*, edited by R. T. Woods, 219–252. Wiley, Chichester.

Yost, E.B., Beutler, L.E., Corbishley, M.A. and Allender, J.R. (1986) *Group Cognitive Therapy: a Treatment Approach for Depressed Older Adults*. Psychology Practitioner Guide, London; Pergamon, New York.

Yesavage, J.A., Brink, T.L. and Rose, T.L. (1983) Development of a geriatric depression scale: a preliminary report. *Journal of Psychiatric Research*, **17**, 37–49.

The role of the nurse in the assessment, diagnosis and management of depression in older people

9

Martin Neal, Philip Hughes and Maggie Bell

Introduction

In order to provide comprehensive assessment and to meet the complex care needs of the older person, multi-professional teamwork is essential. Within this team nurses have a valuable and unique contribution to make. The challenge for nurses, is defining this distinctive role and articulating it to our colleagues.

McKenna (1997) notes the 'hidden' aspects of nursing which include detailed assessment, identification of physical, psychological and social needs, monitoring and evaluation. Nurses are the principal occupational group to provide 24 hour care, they often have the highest level of direct contact with patients, therefore their observations in a number of contexts and the recording of such, contributes significantly towards the team's understanding of the patient and the formulation of a holistic care plan. In this context the nurse provides the continuity of care and acts as information broker.

One definition of mental health nursing (Dexter and Walsh 1995) states that

> mental health nursing is the practice of caring for people who have mental illness, potentiating their independence and restoring their dignity. In order to fulfil this arduous occupation, the mental health nurse must possess a sound knowledge base and the requisite skills of good nursing practice. The ideal nurse must be able to look after the physical needs of the client and understand the social and psychological function of the individual, both normal and abnormal, and have the necessary ability to direct her skills appropriately.

Whilst fully supporting the above description we would argue that those aspects form the basis of the nurse's role, are fundamental to good working practice are not to be seen as a potentially unattainable 'ideal'.

In the review of mental health nursing (Department of Health 1994), chaired by Professor Tony Butterworth, a number of important issues were identified:

Key principles of mental health nursing

- The principle of choice for people who use services and their carers needs to be fully established as a basis for the practice of mental health nursing.
- The work of mental health nurses rests on their relationship with people who use mental health services and that this relationship should have value to both partners.
- It is a fundamental right that 'people who use mental health services can expect to receive skilled, sensitive, professional support from competent mental health nurses'.

Whilst we endorse all of these principles within this chapter, it is the final statement relating to skill and knowledge which has been the focus of attention for professional guidance.

The Royal College of Nursing (1997) notes that 'all older people with mental health needs are entitled to have their care needs assessed by skilled Registered Nurses'. Within this work they go on to describe the knowledge skills and experience of the nurse stating that 'Registered Nurses have:

- Broad empirical knowledge, which derives from the fundamental sciences from which nursing is synthesised (such as psychology, physiology, sociology), from nursing knowledge and research or from that of an allied profession (such as medicine, pharmacology or ergonomics).
- Tacit knowledge which enable nurses to act on hunches or intuition and engage in holistic problem solving. This can be particularly significant in unpacking the complexities of change in the health of older people.
- Broad experience which enables nurses to recognise similarities in patterns of events from previous encounters with older people. Registered Nurses recognise subtle changes in an older person's health status, understand the potential consequences, and then act appropriately.'

The *skills* that Registered Nurses use in everyday practice include

- Observation skills, such as recognizing significant changes and formulating options.
- Psychosocial skills, such as inter-personal communication with residents, their families and colleagues. Nurses also have supporting, encouraging, facilitatory and counselling skills. They are skilled in reflecting, challenging and giving constructive feedback.
- Psycho-motor skills, such as those required to operate equipment.

Nursing assessment

Assessment forms the foundation for identifying needs and interventions for care and contributes to effective and timely discharge planning. It is therefore essential that it be undertaken in a systematic and collaborative manner, working in partnership with the patient, their significant others and the multi-professional team (see Case History, 9.1a). Assessment is an ongoing and continuous process, building a picture over time of an individual and their world. It is important to recognize the difference between the baseline and comprehensive assessment, as the former often provides only a 'snapshot' which can be misleading.

What do we need to know?

The main areas of consideration for mental health nursing assessment are:

- Identifying the norm for an individual and what is happening now, and
- the broad categories of mood, cognitive/emotional state and behaviour.
- Identifying and managing risk.

Case History 9.1a

Mrs Marion P, aged 71 was referred by her GP to the Day Treatment Services for assessment. Her problems included generalized loss of energy and poor appetite in addition to rheumatoid arthritis and hypertension. She also had pneumonia in 1988. There was no history of past psychiatric history and no family history of psychiatric problems.

She was born in Shropshire and had a normal childhood, leaving school at the age of 15. Initially she worked as a wages clerk. She married at the age of 24 and had six children. She returned to work at 35 as a library assistant. Her husband died suddenly in 1988 following a myocardial infarction. This was a great surprise to Mrs P as he had previously no symptoms of cardiac disease. She retired in 1990. Until recently she was involved in several local groups, especially associated with her church and normally she would describe herself as 'outgoing'.

Mrs P was referred to Day Treatment Services for a period of assessment because of poor appetite for the previous 6 months and generally not looking after herself. She was not enjoying her food and complained that 'everything tastes the same'. She was finding it difficult to keep on top of her housework and this was particularly upsetting for her as she is very house proud. When asked to describe her feelings she said 'it is as if a black cloud is hanging over me' and 'I'm just a bit run down but this is all part of getting old'. Mrs P was not sure how an assessment by Day Treatment Services would help her and was troubled that she 'is wasting everybody's time'.

(A) PERSONAL PROFILE

The aim of this section is to provide a general background and build-up of information about the patient/client prior to their presenting difficulties. Suggested areas to include are:

- Particular reactions to significant life events including marriage, separations, birth of children, death, divorce, etc.
- Education background, type of schooling, further education, etc.
- Employment record and general relationship with colleagues.
- Significant personal relationships and social interaction including marital, sexual, parental and siblings.
- General financial status including any money worries, debts, etc. which may have a bearing.
- Previous mental health, e.g. any previous admissions to hospital, visits to the GP for mental health type problems.
- Previous physical health, e.g. admissions to hospitals, general state of health, etc.
- Relevant family health history which could include, patterns of ill health in family, any significant hereditary type illnesses, any important illness in immediate relatives.
- Spiritual Dimension, assessment should seek to evaluate the significance of the practice of a religious or spiritual discipline (e.g. church membership, meditation, yoga, pacifism) as it relates to social support networks, self-esteem, long-term hopes and expectations, etc.
- Hobbies, interests and leisure activities. How they fill their time.

- Support network – who do they have round them to support them, e.g. friendships, helpful neighbours, formal carers, clubs, associations, etc.

(B) HOME ENVIRONMENT

This section provides a general description of how the person lives and should include aspects which are of particular importance to the client. General areas to consider are:

- Type of accommodation, e.g. house, shared house, hostel, living with others, etc.
- General living situation such as condition of house, local environment, etc. This description should reflect differing points of view including, for example, clients, their families, carers or professionals.
- General amenities in their environment, e.g. closeness of shops, bus routes, health centres, etc.

(C) BACKGROUND TO PRESENTING PROBLEMS (FROM THE PERSPECTIVE OF THE CLIENT/PATIENT)

In this section we are looking for the patient's or client's own perceptions as to how their problems have arisen and developed to their present position. Areas to include are as follows:

- Problems and difficulties as stated by the patient, e.g. what are the things the patient wants to talk about? The initial subjects may not be the most important ones. This section could therefore be added to as the assessment develops.
- Starting point – when do they feel the difficulties first started?
- Ongoing history to present time – how have the difficulties and problems progressed.
- Factors involved – the variables that have contributed to the ongoing difficulties, e.g. living conditions, family/marital conflict, ill health, etc. and the duration of these factors.
- Forms of help already tried – what other means have been tried to resolve the present difficulties, e.g. forms of self help, contact with professional or other caring agencies. How successful was this help?
- Attitudes to admission/referral, e.g. did the patient or client refer themselves? Or has somebody made the referral on their behalf? How do they feel about professionals becoming involved? Or being admitted to hospital?
- What form of help do they think they require, e.g. are there any obvious or immediate things they think can be done to help them, what do they want of us?
- Desirable solution as seen by the patient.

(D) BACKGROUND TO THE PRESENTING PROBLEM (AS SEEN BY OTHERS)

It might be thought that the most obvious source of information is the patient themselves, however in the case of patients who are experiencing depression this is not always possible due to motor retardation, associated psychotic ideation, or the presence of overvalued ideas. Valuable information can be obtained from significant others that have been involved so far, i.e. family, friends, professionals including GP, Health Visitor, CPN, etc. It is important to explain to the patient what information is to be obtained and why. Except where risk is high, others should only be approached with the consent of the patient. Points to include should be:

- Problems and difficulties as seen by others.
- Starting point – when do they feel the problems first started?
- History to present time, e.g. what sorts of things have contributed to the problems continuing or not being resolved and the duration of these factors?
- Attitudes to intervention, e.g. what do they feel about the help that is being offered, are they for the referral or against it? Have they made the referral and do they agree with what is going on?
- Form of help required, e.g. what do they feel needs to be done to resolve the patient's problems?
- Desirable solution as seen by others, e.g. what needs to change and what outcome are they looking for?

Nursing observations

This section includes a major area of the nursing assessment. Therefore, to make it easier it has been subdivided into four sub-categories described below. An example of a nursing assessment is summarized in Case History 9.1b.

(A) DESCRIPTION OF PRESENTING BEHAVIOUR

- It is important to include observations of the patient's behaviour across environmental settings and over a period of time. Their behaviour in relation to the changing nature of the social environment is therefore recorded.
- General behaviour patterns – i.e. discernible idiosyncrasies. For example, is the patient predictable or impulsive, organized or disorganized, overactive or retarded?
- Verbal and non-verbal communications – i.e. the pattern and content of communication, e.g. the speed, tone and fluency of speech, the subject matter and topics covered, their relevance and appropriateness to the situation in question, etc.
- Social interaction and attitudes to others – i.e. the nature and manner of the interactions. For example, is the patient assertive, aggressive, stubborn, competitive or humble, conforming and submissive to group pressures?

Case History 9.1b

Initial nursing assessment

Behaviour: On her first visit she spoke little to other patients but responded to questions from staff. She did not initiate conversation and had little eye contact. She frequently sat with hands clasped in her lap.

Affect: There was evidence of low mood, social withdrawal, poor eye contact, closed posture and subjective feeling of being 'down'.

Thought: She initially found it difficult to concentrate during the interview and on several occasions asked for questions to be repeated. She was also slow to respond. She participated minimally in the group social activity and returned to the dining area after 20 minutes.

Memory/Orientation: She said she felt 'very forgetful' but on objective examination no cognitive problems were apparent.

Perception/Cognition: There were no perceptual problems but impaired concentration was evident.

Communication: Her speech was slow speech and this combined with poor eye contact impaired her ability to communicate.

Physical health: She has rheumatoid arthritis, raised blood pressure, wears spectacles and complained of poor sleep. She said she only get 4 hours sleep per night, usually waking early between 4.00 and 5.00 a.m.

Elimination: No expressed problems.

Hygiene: She did not described having any problems. However, her nails and the skin on the back or her neck were dirty. In addition, her clothes were crumpled and some food stains were present. Her hair was slightly greasy and unkempt.

Weight: She has lost approximately 6[space]kg over the previous 2 months.

Mobility: She did not describe problems but she walks with a slight limp. She also occasionally seemed to be experiencing pain in her foot.

Skin: All pressure points intact, but her skin appeared very fragile.

Physical and social environment: She lives alone in privately owned house. This is a large house with four bedrooms and a large garden. It has been the family home for 38 years. She has five daughters and one son and has a good relationship with all of them but she has little contact with them because they live away. There is, however, frequent telephone contact with her family. She has been not told them that she is having health problems because 'they're busy and have enough worries of their own'. She has several close friends but has seen little of them recently as she has not been going out.

Leisure activity: A range of valued activities were identified including involvement in church groups, cooking, baking, reading and watercolour painting. She has a large garden which she used to enjoy caring for but no longer feels able to manage it. She has not engaged in any valued activity over the last few months and feels it is because of a lack of energy and to some extent joint pain.

Does the patient initiate conversations and show an interest in others? Or is the patient passive and withdrawn?

- Personal appearance, i.e. type of dress, whether there are signs of poor self image/self neglect through their appearance and general presentation.
- Personal hygiene, i.e. whether they need help in maintaining their personal hygiene, etc.

- Life skills, i.e. general abilities to perform tasks which would include budgeting, domestic chores, cooking, shopping, interaction with the public, etc.

(B) COGNITIVE/EMOTIONAL STATE

This can be seen as the nursing interpretation of the presenting behaviours as well as observations of the emotional state. Areas to include would be:

- Insight and understanding.
- Level of consciousness and awareness.
- Concentration and attention span.
- General interests in their surroundings and environment.
- Orientation to time, place and person.
- Description of mood and appropriateness to situation.
- Normal way of showing emotions, i.e. how do they express themselves and show their anger, pleasure, sadness, etc.
- Memory, i.e. short-term loss, long-term difficulties, confabulation, etc.
- Thought content, i.e. evidence of delusions, thought blocking, poverty of thought, thought insertion/withdrawal, flight of ideas, etc.
- Perceptions of self, i.e. self image, self awareness, how do they see themselves, what do they think of themselves, etc.
- Problems solving ability – e.g. is the patient able to make a realistic self-appraisal of problems or not? Is the patient able to decide upon a realistic course of action in dealing with such problems? What are their motivations to solve such problems?
- Coping skills, e.g. can the patient identify the kind of thoughts and events which trigger feelings of anxiety/tension, anger/frustration, insecurity/unhappiness, etc.? What kinds of thoughts and activities are personally relaxing and pleasurable to the patient, and how are these utilized in personal strategies for relieving distressing thoughts and feelings?

The patient's perspective on their illness is also important and an example of this is summarized in Case History 9.1c.

(C) PHYSICAL ASSESSMENT

Consideration of all factors affecting the older person is essential as mental health problems are not found in isolation from physical and sensory conditions and impairment may contribute significantly to the feeling of health and well-being and to realistic implementation of care plans. Comments should include in this section:

- Known physical illness, signs and symptoms, any ongoing treatments being received.
- General physical condition, e.g. level of fitness and general health.
- Sensory integration, sight/hearing, awareness of pressure, assistive devices used. Co-ordination and dexterity.
- Sleep pattern, e.g. any disturbance in sleep pattern, and if so, when, what time of day, and for how long?

Case History 9.1c

Patients perception of problems/needs

Mrs P initially repeated her view that her problems are just part of getting old. She appeared to feel hopeless about this, and unable to do anything to improve how she felt. She was prompted to talk more about her life history. She was born in Shropshire where she went to school and remembers having a happy childhood, enjoying school and having a wide circle of friends. She was disappointed to have to leave school at 15 and would have liked to have continued her education. She initially worked as a wages clerk and found this 'OK' but not challenging. She married at the age of 24 and her husband then got a job in West Yorkshire where she has lived ever since. She returned to work when she was 40 years old when her youngest child had started school. There was some opposition to this from her husband but as she was feeling bored and frustrated at home, he eventually agreed. She got a job as a library assistant which she continued with until retiring in 1990. She was very happy in this job, she found it interesting and had lots of social contact. Until recently she has continued to maintain contact with some of her ex-colleagues.

On retirement began to develop a very active social lifestyle with lots of involvement in church groups and leisure activities. She did not want to talk about her husband stating 'some things are better left alone' and due to her distress this was not explored further (at this point).

- Nutrition, i.e. weight, appetite, diet, appropriate food for physical condition, preferred meal times, eating patterns, portions and special needs/preferences.
- Elimination, e.g. general bowel/bladder habits, determine normal pattern and current pattern. Continence, constipation, ability to find and use toilet, any intervention needed, prompting, level of supervision, continence aids, abnormalities in excreta.
- Libido, ability to recognize and perform desired sexual activities in contextually appropriate ways.
- Hygiene, self care, ability to initiate getting washed and dressed including any intervention needed, prompting level of supervision required, bathing, shaving, cleaning teeth.
- Mobility, e.g. level of mobility, any particular problems in mobility, can they climb stairs, can they walk unaided, need help to stand or raise self and standing tolerance, mobility aids used and moving and handling techniques/equipment required.
- Skin integrity, existing wounds, rashes, dryness, and infestation. This should include pressure sore risk assessment.
- Baseline observations of blood pressure, temperature, pulse, weight and urinalysis must be undertaken and recorded, local guidelines and structures determining when this is done and by whom, will direct practice.

(D) SOCIAL INTERACTION PATTERN

As part of the assessment, the nurse should attempt to record any significant social interaction patterns in order to gain greater insight into the presenting difficulties.

These should include:

- Degree of contact with family members and friends, i.e. marital partner, children, parents, etc.
- Significant relationships within the family and social environment, i.e. closer to one than other, who do they have the most contact and involvement with?
- Problematic orientations, e.g. evidence of any obvious conflict or stresses, the individual's social competence.
- What is the level of insight and understanding/empathy, etc. of those identified as significant by the patient, e.g. who is most concerned, who visits, who is taking the responsibility for the identified patient, what are the attitudes of those involved to the patients presenting difficulties?, etc.
- Social networks and participation in activities, both previously and currently.
- Spiritual and cultural needs – e.g. the observation of any cultural or religious requirement preferences.

How do we get this information?

Given we have identified earlier that nursing staff are often in the best position to gather the most complete picture about an individuals mental and physical health it begs the question, what are the best ways in which to gather the information that will facilitate the most effective care being delivered? The key to gathering information is in the formulation of a strategy that ensures that that which is being collated is relevant to the problem being addressed. It also considers the importance of the material in relation to the whole. The information that is identified needs to be collected from a number of sources in order to collate and verify the most accurate picture of both the presenting problems and progress that is being made following any intervention that is undertaken.

In the case of patients who have a planned admission, any previous notes, both medical and nursing should be obtained prior to the admission. In the case of the patients who are admitted as an emergency it is essential that this occurs at the earliest opportunity in order to determine such factors as risk, and to identify previous interventions that were found to be effective.

The more sources of information that are utilized in the collation of any plan of care the higher the likelihood of the information obtained being valid, thereby leading to more effective care.

It is important that during the information gathering process, there is not repetition or duplication of material collected. To this end the establishment of mechanisms that identify when, how and by whom this information is to be collected, greatly enhance the overall efficiency of data collection. Such mechanisms include protocols, policies and increasingly the use of integrated care pathways.

Sources of information

Information can be gathered from the following sources:

- interviews with the patient;
- interviews with significant others;
- observation;
- the use of standardized assessment tools; and
- discussion with other members of the nursing team.

Interviews with the patient

The following areas should be considered in interviewing the patient:

- **Intra-personal:** how the depression has affected the individual from their perspective
- **Inter-personal:** how their depression has affected their relationships with others
- **Extra-personal:** how their depression has affected their relationships with society as a whole (Neuman 1980).

Interviews with significant others

In addition to gaining information about the patients current problems the perception of others can serve to provide useful insights into patterns of behaviour prior to the onset of their depression, and how they were coping with the external world.

Observation

It might be argued that much of the essence of nursing is *observation*. Observation can occur on a formal and informal level. Benner (1984) identifies that the concept of being in another's presence; 'presencing' is an essential part of part of nursing. In order to do this one has to establish rapport, only by being present with another can rapport be established. During this time the nurse is also in an ideal position to observe and formulate opinions about the condition or progress that the patient is making.

It is worthy to note that the lack of observation and the failure of nurses to engage in activities and relationships with patients has been a recurrent criticism within recent reports by the Mental Health Act Commission (1999). Observation can also take the form of standardized observation assessment tools.

The use of standardized assessment tools

There are numerous tools that are available to measure a variety of aspects relating to the features that are presented by depressed patients. It is worth considering the following before utilizing such tools:

- Are they well validated?
- Do the tools have good inter-rater reliability?
- Does the organization have the publisher's permission to use the tool?
- Have the staff using the tool been trained in its use and interpretation?

Such tools can be of use in determining such things as level of depression and anxiety, sleep. Assessment tools that are used within the context of multi-disciplinary teams should have clearly defined tasks and identify the timing of these in order that information is not overlooked or replicated. All those using assessment tools should be *au fait* as to why they are undertaking any activity that is expected of them.

Discussion with other members of the nursing team

The presence of other trained nurses who can contribute to the evaluation of the suitability, relevance and effectiveness of the care that is being delivered should not be overlooked. The use of reflection with colleagues as to the accuracy of the assessment of patients can help prevent the development of tunnel vision. It serves to provide a means of remaining impartial and professional whilst ensuring that the patients' need are met.

What do we do with the information we have gathered?

Having gathered information from a variety of sources the next task has to be the organization of it into a format that is of value. If one draws upon knowledge management terminology, it is the turning of tacit information (bits of factual information that have potential use but that are not being utilized to their full capacity) into explicit knowledge (knowledge that is based upon the utilization of explicit information turning it into a format that can be used in decision making and practice).

Given the current climate and drive towards clinical governance and the move to deliver more effective and efficient clinical practice based upon the better use of knowledge; it is fitting that such an approach becomes the norm (Department of Health 1998).

Ward (1992) identifies that the purpose of assessment is the production of nursing diagnosis, or clinical diagnoses. It the purpose of these diagnoses to generate clear, simple and specific statements that identify client's problems or as Mayers (1983) observes, potential problems. In order to do this the nurse must utilize both inductive and deductive thinking, as illustrated in Figure 9.1.

Having identified the process for decision making the nurse has then to consider how to identify and prioritize those areas of patient need. There is consistent agreement amongst many authors that the work of Maslow (1970) has much to offer. Various authors have provided models of how Maslow's original hierarchy of needs might be interpreted in the field of nursing practice.

Figure 9.2, demonstrates Maslow's hierarchy with two added categories of

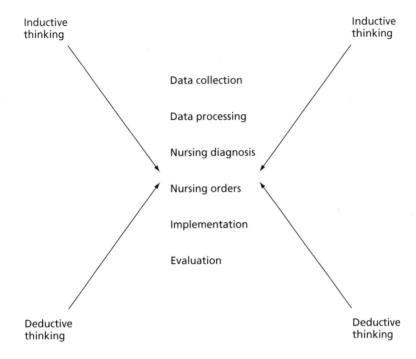

Figure 9.1 The use of inductive and deductive thinking in nursing practice (from La Monica 1983, cited in La Monica 1985).

creative and cognitive needs (adapted from Hersey and Blanchard (1982) and supported by Ward (1992)).

Catherman (1990) identifies that those needs identified at levels 5, 6 and 7 are achieved through the individual being able to successfully achieve their initial needs and their experience determines their ability to consequently self-actualize. The nurse does not directly have the ability to influence these areas and therefore should focus on helping patients achieve those areas that they have the ability too, namely levels 1 to 4 (Ward 1992). An important dimension not emphasized in this hierarchy is the need to 'synergize' – to live and work in a social context with others.

Setting the priorities of nursing interventions

Marks-Maran *et al.* (1988) identify that priority setting is a highly sophisticated exercise. They observe that historically the priorities that have been identified are those that are identified as being important to parties or institutions other than the patient. To this end they advocate the use of the following process to help prioritize those nursing or clinical diagnoses that require

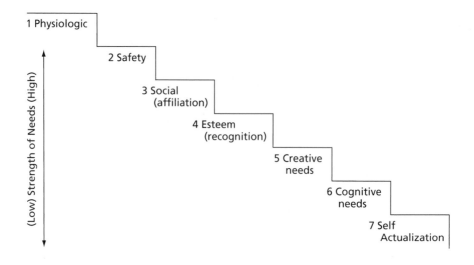

Figure 9.2 Hierachy of needs (adapted from Hersey and Blanchard 1982 and Ward 1992).

immediate and longer-term action (Maran-Marks *et al.* 1988). The process for identifying priorities for nursing activities is described in Figure 9.3.

The use of the following approach can greatly enhance the nurse's understanding of how the individual is experiencing their depression at any time. In the interview with the patient and in the planning of subsequent care the following headings can help this process (**SOAPIE**; adapted from Weed 1970):

S **Subjective:** how the patient feels about their depression and the impact it has had upon them.

O **Objective:** the nurse's perception of the patient's depression based upon the information they are given and the signs that they observe.

A **Assessment:** the formulation of a patient's needs in relation to the above.

P **Planning:** the interventions that are required in order to address these needs.

I **Implementation:** how the interventions identified should be implemented in order to address the patient's needs arising out the assessment.

E **Evaluation:** the evaluation of the effectiveness of any interventions made in relation to the patient's identified needs. At this point the process begins again with the patient being involved in the evaluation process.

The inclusion of the implementation and evaluation stages has meant that this process lends itself well to being integrated with approaches such as the nursing process, primary nursing and the use of nursing models.

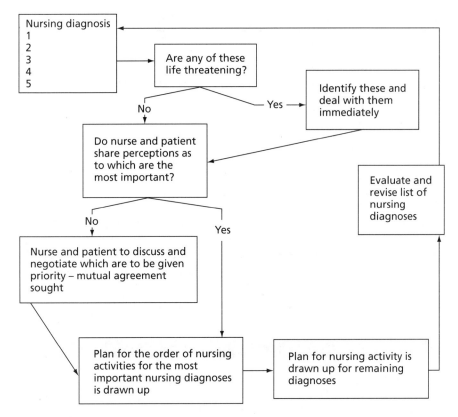

Figure 9.3 The process for identifying priorities for nursing activities.

The use of clinical or nursing diagnosis is a formal way of ensuring the following:

- a means to becoming totally aware of patient problems, or potential problems;
- identification of the causes; and
- identification of behaviours that arise as a result of these problems (Mark-Maran *et al*. 1988).

The real skill in care planning is firstly the ability to identify problems and their causes, then to place them in an order that prioritizes them whilst at the same time not losing sight of the patient's wishes and desires. Ward (1992) identifies that there should be no more than five nursing actions identified in any care plan; the care plan providing a prioritized 'minimum' set of actions that must occur with additional nursing action being delivered whenever nursing resources allow.

The introduction of electronic patient notes and single patient case notes has had a great impact on the organization and availability of information about patient care needs that are available to the multi-disciplinary team. Ward (1992) identifies that the following should be born in mind when

Table 9.1. Points to consider when creating nursing care plans.

1. Care plans should be patient orientated.
2. Objectives should be realistic.
3. Objectives should be provable.
4. They should be quantitative, stating explicitly expectations of any actions that are to occur.
5. They should be succinct, whilst at the same time not becoming so reduced as to become meaningless.
6. They should contain time limits, and contain both short- and long-term objectives.
7. Objectives should have a logical sequence that relates to the achievement of any outcomes that are described.

prescribing nursing care. This list serves to provide a useful aide-mémoire when creating nursing care plans (Table 9.1).

It is only by the use of a consistent and systematic approach to care planning that relevant care be achieved. To this end the adoption of frameworks that are agreed and monitored by nursing teams can only serve to help promote better nursing practice. There are a myriad of potential frameworks that can be utilized, what is essential is that the one chosen has been so because it fits the needs of the patient group who are being cared for.

Case History 9.1d

Perhaps the most significant loss for Mrs P was the death of her husband. From the initial assessment one can only speculate about the impact this has had on Mrs P. Further exploration is required as rapport and the relationship between patient and nurse develops. It would be worth considering exploring the following areas that might have resulted from the death of her husband:

- reduced confidence;
- loss of friendship and companionship;
- loneliness;
- loss or reduction in emotional and physical support;
- loss of sexual relationship; and
- loss of practical support, e.g. financial management.

Once all the information has been collected it is helpful to produce an *Initial Assessment Summary* and an example of this is summarized in Table 9.2. Further information about Mrs P is summarized in Case History 9.1d.

How can we achieve the goals?

Here we must explore what it is that nurses do to or with people which:

1. Help the older person with a depressive illness; and

Table 9.2. Initial Assessment Summary.

Physical	Psychological	Social	Environmental	Spiritual
• Mobility exacerbated	• Concentration	• Church activities	• Maintenance of garden	• Church attendance and
• Dexterity by pain	• Self-worth and value	• Group leisure activities	• Maintenance of house	• Participation in worship, etc.
• Visible evidence of ageing	• Positive outlook and thought	• Social network		• Access to spiritual guidance/
• Self-care skills	• Positive feedback	• Family contact		• Support
• Independence		• Occupation (paid or other)		
• Purposeful physical activities		• Contact with ex-colleagues		
• Appetite and weight loss				
• Sleep				
• Energy				

2. Is distinct from that which a patient would receive from any other professional.

There are a number of ways in which the nurse can work with and for the patient to achieve the goals identified in the care plan. These can be broadly categorized into six areas:

- implementing care plans – the level or intensity of intervention;
- care management/co-ordination;
- information giving;
- supportive activities;
- enabling activities; and
- therapeutic activities.

This is not intended to be an exhaustive list of all the possible interventions a nurse may have to offer nor should it be seen as a blueprint for all nursing activity with older people suffering from depression. However, we would suggest that most activities that a nurse would engage in to help the patient achieve their goals would fall into one of the above categories.

The key factor in all of these categories, indeed all the work that a nurse conducts with a patient and more often than not the key factor in success or failure, is the nature and strength of the relationship between nurse and patient. Chinn and Kramer (1995) identify the interpersonal relationships between the nurse and other individuals as 'the core element of the helping process that is the basis of nursing'. The skill of the nurse is in our opinion best demonstrated in developing a relationship where trust and empathy exist for the purpose of helping the patient and that there is clarity about the purpose and limits of that relationship. There is a risk in developing such relationships that they become friendship with one or both parties losing track of the specific purpose of the relationship. The UKCC (1998) point out that 'A client may develop a degree of psychological dependence upon you during a professional relationship. You must be aware of this and the risks it presents to the working relationship'. This can be guarded against by the setting out of shared goals and likely length of the involvement at an early stage, the use of contracts that outline the expectations and intentions of each party. Such contracts would also include issues around access to and the sharing of and disclosure of information.

Implementing care plans

Care plans should be written in collaboration with patients and when appropriate their carers and this process of negotiation should continue at the point of implementation. The care plans provide the structure for interventions based upon the needs identified in the assessment, they are the basis for guiding care, providing continuity of care where different nurses are involved with one patient, and for communication to other professions and interested parties. The care plan will also ideally provide the patient with a record for reference and clarity of purpose, it can be a documented basis for the contract between nurse and patient. The 'named nurse' will write the care plans and act on and/or oversee the implementation of the care plans.

The interventions offered may include one-to-one work with an individual, group work, problem-solving exercises and practical support. The level of intensity will depend upon the severity of the sufferer's problems and the extent to which they are disabled by them. Orem (1995) offers a framework for nursing interventions based on the normal pattern of a patient's life.

Care management/co-ordination

One role that nurses invariably perform for patients but until recently has had little recognition, especially by nursing theorists, is that of care manager/co-ordinator. The nurse has, alongside other professionals, often taken on the responsibility for organizing the input of other professions and workers to the care and treatment of their patients, a role that has become more formalized in the form of the 'Care Programme Approach' (Department of Health 1990). The National Framework for Mental Health (Department of Health 1999b) and Effective Care Co-ordination in Mental Health Services – Modernising the Care Programme Approach (Department of Health 1999a) give further guidance on the role of Care Co-ordinator and policy advice to Health Trusts, Authorities and Local Authorities about the integration of care programme approach and care management. All this emphasizes the need to be proactive in discharge planning and care co-ordination, to actively 'network', seeking knowledge about and support for, each patient and actively reviewing the care packages provided. Although the National Service Framework approach excludes older people, further guidance is expected in the National Service Framework for older people, due to be published in 2000.

Supporting activities

Many of the informal but nevertheless valuable (to the patient) activities, fall into this category. They can range from what Benner (1984) describes as 'presencing' – the act of just being with someone at a time of deep emotional turmoil or trauma, to practical tasks such as arranging for the care of a pet during a period of hospitalization. Supportive activities are performed as and when required often on the spur of the moment but also they can be planned. It is important to recognize that these activities should, as their title suggests, support the patient's recovery and not contribute to a disempowering erosion of skills and confidence and loss of independence, which can occur in people who suffer from debilitating depressive illnesses.

In support of such activities there should be a care plan that identifies such actions as planned activities in response to identified needs. When medication is necessary the nurse can have an important role in supporting and helping the unmotivated patient to understand the need for such treatment, in providing appropriate supervision and in monitoring progress and side-effects.

Information giving

Knowledge is power and equally a lack of knowledge, especially when one is feeling vulnerable, is likely to contribute to a feeling of dependence upon anyone who is in the position of helping. As with any serious illness, when one becomes depressed there is a natural desire on the part of the sufferer and their family or supporters for information about the illness, possible causes, treatments and potential side-effects, likely duration, what can be done to help alleviate symptoms, and what to expect from the professionals involved.

There are two issues to consider in this section, firstly the nature of information that will be useful and secondly the ways in which such information can be given. The most immediate information that sufferers seek is often related to possible help and treatment to alleviate the symptoms and the likely duration of their current state – 'when will I start to feel better?'. The nurse must make some judgement as to the most appropriate information for each patient dependent on that patient's circumstances and the information that each individual patient seeks. Unfortunately there is a tendency for all sufferers to be handed a standard leaflet on depression as a matter of course with little further consideration of their information needs.

Aside from information relating to the illness, the individual may well have a variety of information needs depending on circumstances e.g. relating to benefits, housing, bereavement, social activities and groups, etc. Such information is predominantly in the form of written literature at present, however face to face discussion and explanation of the material is important wherever possible – when depressed an individuals ability to concentrate and read is often severely impaired. Information is becoming more available in audio or videotape format and many people now own the technology to make use of these sources although there may be a cost implication.

Negotiation should also take place as to whether the nurse seeks and provides the information or helps the sufferer to identify and satisfy his or her own information needs. In most situations there will be a compromise between these two examples moving progressively towards the second as the sufferer's condition improves.

Enabling activities

In each of the activities already covered there are examples of enabling activities. An enabling activity can be any activity that has the intention of helping an individual to improve their own situation. Enabling has been described in the context of people with learning difficulties as the encouragement of free choice in a non-directive way within a caring and supportive environment (Haggar and Hutchinson 1991).

Such activities include problem solving, which includes the identification and prioritization of problems, and the learning life skills. Helping a patient to recognize and prioritize those issues that he/she identifies as problems can help him/her to gain some control or feeling of control, over these issues that otherwise can appear to form into an unmanageable mass. The skill of the nurse is to estimate when an older person suffering from depression is able to engage in this activity.

Many older people become depressed following significant changes in their lives such as retirement or the loss of a partner. The result of such events may lead to a change in situation that requires the learning of everyday skills of life such as cooking, financial management, household management, etc. The nurse can play a key role in enabling a person to develop or re-visit these skills as part of their care for them.

Therapeutic activities

The therapeutic activities that the nurse may engage in with a patient will of course depend on the nature of the problems faced. They range from various styles of counselling, structured approaches to the management of anxiety (which often accompanies depression) or anger, through to cognitive behavioural approaches to the treatment of depression.

Whilst exposed to most, if not all these modes of treatment in their basic training, the psychiatric nurse is not trained to a level of competency in any of them although many do gain such qualifications subsequently. The lack of such qualifications does not necessarily rule out these approaches as therapeutic options unless a referral is made to a specialist worker. It is possible for the nurse to utilize these 'tools' with the appropriate level of supervision, indeed it is vitally important that a nurse receives supervision from a qualified and skilled practitioner in whichever approach is being adopted.

The experience of using a variety of therapeutic approaches is important in developing a range of tools in each nurse's tool box, however these should only be developed in relationships where the over riding purpose is to benefit the individual patient.

Evaluation

The evaluation of a patient's care should be informal and ongoing, as well as structured and periodic. The evaluation should principally focus upon a re-assessment of the patient and their situation to enable discussion about further options and decisions about the next steps to be taken. This establishes a process which Ward (1992) describes as 'dynamic' and 'never-ending', however La Monica (1985) outlines a wider concept which includes the evaluation of carers abilities and the effectiveness of leadership style in the implementation of care.

It is an opportunity to evaluate the effectiveness of the therapeutic interventions offered and to reflect on the learning that has taken place. These can be done with the patient, in the multi-disciplinary team setting using the care programme approach as the vehicle and in clinical supervision. An evaluation of the team's performance may also be indicated to enable team practices to be shaped in the light of practical experiences.

All of this is pertinent to the treatment and care of the individual patient as it is a comprehensive way of ensuring that care continues to focus on the patient's needs and their own goals, and that practice is shaped and guided by evidence of experience and outcome. It also gives the opportunity to consider the widest range of evidence based therapeutic options.

Key points

- This chapter has sought to clarify the valuable and unique nursing contribution to the treatment of the older person suffering from depression.
- This contribution may stand alone, but will be most effective as an element of a co-ordinated inter-disciplinary team approach.
- We acknowledge the unique contribution of all professionals and recognize the benefits that a complementary team approach can offer to patient care.
- The high level of direct patient contact that nursing staff provide facilitates the development of effective therapeutic relationships, it is this we believe that underpins the quality of nursing care of depressed patients.
- The nature of nursing older people who may have complex needs affecting various dimensions of their lives, demands a synthesis of knowledge, skill and experience to develop the advanced level of competence that is required to deliver truly holistic care.
- If the contribution of nursing is to be recognized on equal terms with other health care professionals in meeting the challenges of the clinical governance agenda it must be able to demonstrate a body of knowledge that is based upon critical appraisal skills and evidence-based practice.

References

Benner, P. (1984) *From Novice to Expert: Excellence and Power in Clinical Nursing Practice.* Addison Wesley, Reading, Massachusetts.

Cathermam, A. (1990) Biopsychosocial nursing assessment; a way to enhance care plans. *Journal of Psychosocial Nursing and Mental Health Services,* **28**, 31–33.

Chinn, P. L. and Kramer, M.K. (1995) *Theory and Nursing, A Systematic Approach,* 4th edn. Mosby, St Louis.

Department of Health (1990) *The Care Programme for People with a Mental Illness Referred to the Specialist Psychiatric Services.* HC (90) 23/LASSL (90) 11, DH.

Department of Health (1994) *Working in Partnership.* Report of the Mental Health Nursing Review Team, HMSO, London.

Department of Health (1998) First Class Service – Quality in the New NHS. HMSO, London.

Department of Health (1999a) *Effective Care Co-ordination in Mental Health – Modernising the Care Programme Approach.* HMSO, London.

Department of Health (1999b) *The National Framework for Mental Health Services.* HMSO, London.

Dexter, G. and Walsh, M. (1995*) Psychiatric Nursing Skills: A Patient-Centred Approach,* 2nd edn. Chapman and Hall, London.

Haggar, L.E., and Hutchinson, R.B. (1991) Snoezelen: an approach to the provision of a leisure resource for people with profound and multiple handicaps. *Mental Handicap,* **19**, 51–55.

Hersey, P. and Blanchard, K. (1982) *Management of Organisational Behaviour; Utilising Human Resources,* 4th edn. Prentice-Hall, Englewood Cliffs, NJ.

La Monica, E.L. (1983) *Nursing Leadership and Management: An Experimental Approach.* Wadsworth Health Sciences Division, Belmont.

La Monica, E.L. (1985) *The Humanistic Nursing Process,* Wadsworth Health Sciences Division, Belmont.

Marks-Maran, D.J., Docking, S.P. , Maunder, T. and Scott, J. (1988) *Skills for Care Planning A Guide for Teaching the Nursing Process.* Scutari Press, London.

Maslow, A. (1970) *Motivation and Personality,* 2nd edn. Harper and Row, New York.

Mayers, M. (1983) *A Systematic Approach to the Nursing Care Plan,* 3rd edn. Appleton–Century–Crofts, Norwalk, CT.

McKenna, H. (1997) *Nursing Theories and Models.* Routledge, London.

Mental Health Act Commission (1999) *The 8th Biennial Report, 1977–1999.* Stationery Office Publications, London.

Neuman, B. (1980) The Betty Neuman Health-care systems model: a total person approach to patient problems. In *Conceptual Models for Nursing Practice,* 2nd edn, edited by J. Riehl and C. Roy. Appleton-Century-Crofts, New York.

Orem, D.E. (1995) *Nursing Concepts of Practice,* Mosby, St Louis.

Royal College of Nursing (1997) *How Nurses Can Help You; a RCN Guide for Older People and their Families.* RCN, London.

UKCC (1998) *Guidelines for Mental Health and Learning Disabilities Nursing,* London.

Ward, M.F. (1992) *The Nursing Process in Psychiatry.* Churchill Livingstone, Edinburgh

Weed, L. (1970) 'Medical Records, Medical Education and Patient Care.' Cleveland: Press, Western Reserve University.

The contribution of the occupational therapist to the assessment, diagnosis and treatment of depression in old age

Gail Mountain

Introduction

According to the Department of Health (1997a), major depression affects between 2 and 4% of older people, with a further 10–20% experiencing less severe forms of the illness. Severity is exacerbated by poor rate of detection, even when individuals are already in receipt of health and social care (Banerjee 1993).

Pharmacological treatment of depression is effective but beyond this, professionals and informal carers can struggle to find other solutions to the problems of older people with depression. For some, drugs alone will be all that is needed, particularly if the illness is detected early enough. However, for those with more pervasive, complex problems, their needs may not be satisfied by pharmacological treatments alone, necessitating referral to a range of other professionals and continuing support from a wide care network.

Depression may follow physical illness, the erosion of physical capabilities, and the effects of life events like bereavement and loss of role. There are also a number of individuals who experience depression during their lives, with the illness extending into older age. It is therefore simplistic to think that there is a definitive solution to what is an extremely complicated area of work. Taking this into account, this chapter will describe how occupational therapists can contribute towards the many faceted treatment and care package for older people with depression and their carers. The evidence base which exists in this area is used to identify good practice and to describe how occupational therapy services might develop in the future.

Occupational therapists are primarily concerned with the practicalities of everyday living and the effects of ageing, mental illness, abilities and preferences have all to be considered within this context. The occupational therapist has to be able to respond appropriately to the many and varied daily needs which can result.

Occupation and lifestyle in older age is now considered to provide a contextual framework for the occupational therapy assessment and treatment process.

Occupation and lifestyle

Occupational therapy focuses upon occupation or meaningful doing; a simple statement belying an extremely complex construct. The range of interpretations which can be applied to the term 'occupation' is wide. The American Occupational Therapy Association describe occupations as what people do in their everyday lives (AOTA 1995). These include work, leisure and play.

The importance of occupation underpinned the development of occupational therapy e.g. in the USA the primary concerns of the early occupational therapists centred upon lack of participation in occupations rather than upon diagnosis, disability or loss (Kielhofner and Nicol 1989). Therefore the emphasis was upon holism rather reductionism. This is important given the range of physical, emotional and socio-economic needs that older people and their carers can present with. This belief in the centrality of occupation for human well being has given rise to a number of theories, two being described below.

The theory of human occupation (Kielhofner 1985) describes the human being as an open system which interacts constantly with the external environment. There are three overarching subsystems within the human:

- volition is responsible for choice;

- habituation is concerned with roles and habits; and
- performance is concerned with the ability to do, to learn and to communicate (occupational skills).

Burton (1989) applied the model of human occupation to an examination of the evidence base concerned with normal ageing, drawing out a number of conclusions, some of which do not conform with the stereotypic picture of abilities in older age (see Table 10.1). These findings give important messages for occupational therapy practice. Burton also comments upon the interaction between the older person and the environment. As frailty increases, the environment of the older person diminishes, with an aspect of occupational therapy being to enable the continuing experience of quality of life despite limitations.

The relationship between occupation and health has been made more explicit by Wilcock (1998). She describes three occupational stressors which can mitigate against health: occupational imbalance, occupational deprivation and occupational alienation. Imbalance occurs when an individual experiences too much of the same activity. Deprivation is concerned with lack of opportunities to carry out occupations due to limited opportunity and choice. If a person is unable to meet their occupational needs because of societal factors and the demands which arise from external sources, they may experience occupational alienation. Additionally, Wilcock postulates that all of us are also having to make large occupational adaptations due to factors like technological advances and changing lifestyles.

Lambert (1998) links occupation with lifestyle, describing them as being broadly similar processes. He defines lifestyle as

> the pattern of life adopted by an individual, or group, which is influenced by the resources available to them . . . specific elements include fluid intake, diet, physical

Table 10.1. Summary of findings of review of evidence on normal ageing extracted from a paper by Burton (1989).

Subsystem	Research evidence concerned with normal ageing
Volition	• Little evidence of lowered self-esteem except following sudden loss. • A desire for more control than there is perceived to be. • A tendency to both underestimate and overestimate abilities. • Dwelling on the past is common in depression. • Occupational tasks have different values for individuals. • Leisure interests positively correlate with life satisfaction.
Habituation	• Role loss increases the importance of leisure and social roles. • Institutional routines disrupt the balance of work, rest and leisure. • Maintenance of routines by the individual is important, but there is also evidence of adaptation in response to changing circumstances.
Performance	• Communication skills remain intact except when disrupted by illness. • Perceptual motor skills can slow down. • Learning is important and, while it takes longer, it is not impaired. • Problem solving is good if within the context of familiar situations.

exercise and rest (including sleep, habits, routines and social interactions in which they participate regularly).' (Lambert 1998, pp. 194).

He argues for involvement of occupational therapists in both occupation and lifestyle, and in the encouragement of healthy lifestyles through health promotion and prevention.

Normal adaptations to old age

Older age involves the person adapting to changing circumstances; the success of these adaptations making the experience positive or negative. It is important to understand how this adaptive process is experienced and managed by those who are relatively fit and well, before we can begin to understand the needs of older people who have become depressed. Retirement after a lifetime of employment can be eagerly anticipated or it can be dreaded. Jonsson et al. (1997) conducted a longitudinal study of 32 workers in Sweden to examine how people anticipate retirement. The qualitative study based on the model of human occupation (Kielnhofner 1985) found that most of those interviewed viewed retirement as embracing both positive and negative aspects, with perceptions of work being significant in shaping their views. Women who have spent most of their lives looking after others may enjoy newly found freedom or not know how to spend their time. It may be possible to take opportunities for increased leisure. Alternatively, life interests may become impossible due to infirmity which can accompany increasing age. Stereotypes are difficult to avoid, but their inappropriateness is evident, illustrated in a study of risk-taking in older age (Wynne-Hartley 1991) where a number of *risky activities* undertaken by older people are described. These include skiing, water sports, marathon running and arts and crafts activities which use potentially dangerous equipment.

Studies of occupational adaptation in older age illustrate the diversity of the process and the factors which occupational therapists and other professionals should be alert to. Clark et al. (1996) explored how older people adapt to their lifestyles. They conducted qualitative individual and group interviews with 29 older people living on low incomes in America and residing in the same subsidized accommodation. Analysis revealed 10 life domains including activities of daily living, use of free time, maintenance of mobility and personal finances, with adaptive strategies existing within each. The authors are clear that this typology cannot be generalized as some domains were unique to the population being studied. However they observed that certain of the emergent themes, in particular grave illness, death and spirituality and relationships with others, are often neglected by occupational therapists and others involved in the assessment and treatment of older people.

Ludwig (1997) examined the importance of routine in the lives of seven middle class white older women who were well at the time of study. The qualitative study involved in-depth interviews, autobiographical data collection and observation. He found that the women adapted their routines over time and had willingly relinquished some of their previous life roles. The study identified six implications for occupational therapists:

- Helping older people to link their past to their current lifestyle is important for continuity and to promote a sense of well being.
- When routines can no longer be conducted to a standard which is acceptable to the individual, they are adapted or given up, and then replaced.
- Routine provides a framework which can make the occurrence of certain occupations more likely.
- Health interventions can replace or interrupt longstanding occupation, leading to loss of meaning which can lead to depression.
- The undertaking of occupation which demands more energy should be scheduled into a daily routine which suits the individual.
- Including others in the routine makes the undertaking of the task more likely.

Dickie (1998) discussed the findings of Ludwig's study to draw out guidelines for practice. The importance of listening carefully to the experiences of the person is emphasized. Some people are not able to relinquish roles, particularly if they have wider implications for the family unit, for example caring for others. They are therefore not able to adjust to their changing circumstances. While some people will welcome changes, others will find the giving up of routines difficult and distressing.

The findings from these studies demonstrate the inappropriateness of generalization. They illustrate both the number and complexity of factors which come into play, adjustments which are made readily by some are impossible for others.

The relationship between depression and occupation in old age

> The interplay between depression and occupation is well recognized, Depression does take its toll on occupation . . . the condition is characterized by changes in capacities to engage in goal directed use of time, energy, interest and attention. (Devereaux and Carlson 1992, pp. 175).

Therefore, in addition to the previously described occupational adaptations which all older people have to make, older people who become depressed are faced with additional challenges to their abilities to manage day-to-day tasks. Older women with depression interviewed about their experiences of occupational therapy and specialist mental health services (Mountain 1998) said that they found familiar, necessary tasks like cooking difficult because of the way they were feeling. They used words like *lazy* or *guilty* to try and explain the extent of distress this caused them. Some of those interviewed also expressed the frustrations of trying to maintain independence in the face of physical illness and increasing frailty.

> 'On Sunday, I tried to open a little tin of salmon. I've about five tin openers and I couldn't open it, so I couldn't have salmon for my tea.' (Mrs BP).
> 'I shall be glad when I can go to the shops; it's a nuisance when you can't do your own shopping.' (Mrs KA).

Additionally, the effects of age and infirmity touched other areas of the women's lifestyles and in particular abilities to maintain lifelong interests.

> Mrs HW could not continue her hobbies due to poor hand mobility, 'I love sewing, knitting and crochet but I can't do it any more.'

For some older people living in the community, the emotional implications of losing a lifelong partner will be exacerbated by them being totally unprepared for a single life. In these cases, resulting occupational stressors (using the typology of Wilcock) can either exacerbate or be the root of the depression. Many older women have never learnt to drive, and as a consequence they can find themselves unable to continue with established shopping routines or attendance at social functions. Others will not have participated in the financial management of the household. All those involved in the health and social care of older people will have, at some time, encountered men incapable of cooking simple meals for themselves in widowhood.

Depression combined with a variety of occupational stressors can be experienced by older people living in their own homes. However, it is a far more common occurrence for those who have entered long term care. The incidence of depression in nursing homes and other residential settings is widely acknowledged. It is estimated that around 40% of older people in residential care are depressed (Mann *et al.* 1984). Having to give up one's home and independence will mean that the person will have to relinquish longstanding occupational routines. Depression may also stem from the lack of opportunities for occupation within the residential care environment. Revisit the well-known image of people sitting in chairs around the periphery of a room. The only available stimulation is the television. There is no activity and no conversation. In this situation, the effects of occupational deprivation caused by the environment are all too acute. A small study by Green (1995) examined the outcomes of introducing a programme of activities into a nursing home. Observed and reported benefits on the part of staff, residents and their relatives included enjoyment, animation and relief of boredom. Green noted the willingness by some staff to become involved in the delivery of the activity programme, indicating a potential training role for occupational therapists.

Occupation is central in all our lives, at every stage of life, and wherever we live. As we become older, our occupational needs, lifestyle and abilities change. For those older people who are depressed, there are many factors which can mitigate against the maintenance of an independent, quality lifestyle. This is the backdrop against which the occupational therapist working with older people with depressive illness must respond.

The occupational therapy assessment process

Assessment of the physical and mental well being and functional abilities of older people is a key occupational therapy role. The assessment process can take several forms, for example:

- An interview with the older person and/or their carer using an interview guide.
- Requesting specific information from the older person and/or their carer through a questionnaire applied in an interview situation.
- Structured observation (Finlay 1997) while watching the older person undertaking tasks.
- Measurement of the functional abilities of the older person and/or their participation in activities of daily living through application of assessment instruments.

This assessment process can take place in different settings, for example in:

- acute hospital care;
- other forms of residential setting;
- day care;
- the person's own home.

In common with other health and social care professionals, occupational therapists have traditionally employed their clinical skills to guide the assessment process, with the results of such assessments being in narrative. However, the value of carefully chosen assessment instruments is now recognized. A study by Stewart (1999) compared the use of standardized and non-standardized assessments by occupational therapists working in social services. While the study was small and confined to the activity of one occupational therapist assessing older people referred for minor adaptations to their homes, it raises very relevant questions. Stewart found that use of a non standardized questionnaire limited the ability of the occupational therapist to identify people who were on the margins of frailty and could benefit from further services. A further observation about the value of applying rigorous assessments is that they provide measures or ratings which can then be used as a baseline to examine outcomes of treatment interventions. Objective measurement is difficult if the assessment process is wholly descriptive.

There are many assessment instruments on the market. Important considerations in the choice of assessments include:

- The psychometric properties of the instrument, in particular its reliability and validity.
- The appropriateness of the instrument for assessment of the multiplicity of problems that older people with depression can present with.
- The usability of the instrument; can it be readily applied and analysed; is training required to use it.
- The acceptability of the instrument to the older person and their carer,

including the extent to which it enables the assessment process to be owned by the recipients of the service.

In the case of older people with mental health problems, there can be a multiplicity of presenting problems. Selection of assessments must take into account physical and socio economic factors which may be present, as well as mental health problems. However, it may not be necessary for the occupational therapist to assess all dimensions. If the multi-team is working in a coordinated manner, with shared care planning, information from the assessments of other team members can be drawn together in the development of the overall treatment programme. The occupational therapist should therefore use instruments which provide quality information about occupational needs rather than applying generic measures. Some of the occupational therapy specific assessment instruments which can be used with older people with mental health problems, and their properties are shown in Table 10.2.

While it is important to consider the content of the assessment, the manner in which the assessment is conducted is of equal if not greater significance. A qualitative study of the hospital discharge process by Godfrey and Moore (1996) involved interviewing users and carers, the majority of whom were elderly, about their experiences. Professional influences upon decisions about return home were perceived to be paramount, with the assessment being a test which the user either passed or failed. This belief was expressed clearly by one older lady interviewed during the study by Mountain (1998).

'Well, they said you went in the kitchen to make a meal. If you passed you could go home, but if not you'd have to go and do it again, stay in hospital.'

The research found that those older people who had been referred for occupational therapy assessment only were fearful of both the process and its consequences. The situation did not allow for clarification and reassurance. The importance of aiming to provide treatment following assessment must also be emphasized. Too often, occupational therapists are involved in pre-discharge home assessments. The sole aims of such assessments can be to provide information about risk for the multi-disciplinary team, arrange successful discharge and clear beds (Mountain and Moore 1996). This substantiates the view of the old lady who perceived the assessment as a test. Given the wide range of occupational needs which older people with mental health problems can present with, it is questionable whether they can be satisfied by a one off encounter such as a pre-discharge assessment. However, this should not negate assessment of risk followed by strategies to increase safety. This aspect is discussed in more depth under treatment approaches. Good practice guidelines for assessment are summarized in Table 10.3.

Table 10.2. Occupational therapy specific assessment instruments.

Instrument	Properties	Applicability	Usability	Acceptability/ Suitability
Occupational Performance Interview Kielnhofner et al. (1991)	Reliable and valid for an American population	Provides detailed information through a life history narrative	Need to study manual prior to use and be prepared to translate American terminology. A lot of data to analyse.	Long interview process. May need a number of sessions to complete.
Assessment of Motor and Process Skills (AMPS) Fisher 1995	Standardized internationally and cross-culturally	Measures quality of performance in personal and domestic activities of daily living	Attendance at a recognized training course mandatory	Has been used successfully with older people with mental health problems.
Canadian Occupational Performance Measure (COPM) Law et al. (1994)	Reliable and valid for a Canadian population. Ongoing work to develop COPM for specific English populations	Assesses problems in occupational performance and then measures changes in perception of performance over time	Training recommended and use of training manual. Training video available.	Can be used with older people with mental health problems, but the focus is upon physical limitations
Community Dependency Index Eakin and Baird (1995)	Valid and reliable for community living physically disabled and elderly people	Rates problems in activities of daily living and continence. Can be applied over time to measure outcome	Easily applied rating scale	Measures physical limitations in community settings only, but provides quality information
Comprehensive Occupational Therapy Evaluation (COTE) Brayman and Kirby (1982)	Valid and reliable for people with acute mental health problems in the USA	Provides a structured format for reporting observations during initial assessment. Can then be used to measure change over time.	Not readily obtainable. No special training specified but it would be necessary to study the measure carefully before using it.	Has been successfully used to study occupational therapy outcomes for older people with mental health problems in inpatient hospital care

Table 10.3. Assessment: good practice guidelines.

- Use a range of reliable and valid measures with interview and observation occupational needs and risk factors.
- Remain aware of the anxieties such assessments can generate.
- Determine from the older person what they want and need to be able to do.
- Consider the implications for the older person of undertaking short-term, one-off assessment.
- Give the older person and their carers feedback from the assessment process as a priority and check their perceptions against the results.
- Determine the extent of informal care available and the sustainability of that care.
- Reassess on a regular basis to take account of shifting needs and changes in the care network.

Contributing towards the diagnosis of depression

Occupational therapists are trained to work across health and social care boundaries and are well placed to detect depression in those already in receipt of services. However, as Banerjee (1993) observed, depression and other mental health problems in older age often remain undetected. The majority of occupational therapists who work with older people with mental health problems will become involved when the depressive illness has been confirmed, the older person referred to specialist services and the involvement of the multi-disciplinary team deemed to be appropriate. However, what of those older people who remain undiagnosed? Can occupational therapy help these people to have their needs identified? One of the many benefits of cross boundary service delivery as promoted by current policy is that it facilitates an holistic approach towards the needs of older people. Occupational therapists are trained to work generically and through their observational and assessment skills will be able to identify the existence of decreased levels of occupation in older people in any setting. The next task of is to explore the many reasons for this occurring, for example is it due to:

- Physical ill health.
- Physical frailty leading to decreased ability to undertake occupations.
- A positive choice taken by the person to decrease their levels of activity (evidenced during studies of well older people).
- A consequence of external life influences like social isolation, entering residential care.
- Poor skills, for example as a consequence of being bereaved of a life partner.
- Depression arising from external events like bereavement, a life-threatening illness or poor relationships.
- Depression with no apparent cause.
- Alcoholism.
- Other forms of mental ill health.
- The onset of dementia.

Through treatment of the occupational needs of the older person, the occupational therapist can contribute towards the identification of depression and other forms of mental health problems in the older person. This skill is of particular value if applied in new forms of convalescence and rehabilitation (intermediate care) services for older people which form a bridge between acute and community care (Mountain 1997). In these settings, where rehabilitation is focused upon physical function, it is all too easy to overlook depression. There will also be new opportunities for occupational therapists to be more involved in the early detection of depression in older people as services shift to a primary care focus. Conversely, occupational therapists working in specialist mental health services for older people must explore all the reasons for decreased levels of occupation rather than becoming focused upon mental health problems alone. Through in-depth interviews with older people with depression (Mountain 1998), it became clear that mental health problems were only one facet of the range of problems they were experiencing. A thorough assessment process combined with an interview with the older person and their carer may well highlight a number of reasons for lowered levels of occupation, some of which may indicate a need for practical treatment strategies. Good practice guidelines for diagnosis are summarized in Table 10.4.

Table 10.4. Contributing towards diagnosis: good practice guidelines.

- Look for signs of decreased occupation which cannot be attributed to physical limitations or illness.
- Look beyond the problems presented on referral to consider the totality of the person's lifestyle.
- Allow the older person plenty of time to talk; find out about their previous lifestyle, how satisfied they are with their present life and their aspirations for the future.
- Talk with others the person identifies as being significant to them and determine the support mechanisms they have available to them.

Treatment approaches

Treatment of older people with depression is infrequently reported in the occupational therapy literature, even though there are a growing number of clinical specialists. However those studies which do exist underscore the curative effects of occupation, for example the work of Devereaux and Carlson (1992) and Salo-Chydenius (1994).

Occupational therapy treatment should be geared towards all domains which fall within the sphere of occupation, that is work, leisure and play. For older people this has to take into account the following:

- The results of the assessment.
- What the older person themselves needs to and would like to be able to do.
- Their physical and mental state.

- The risk any situation poses, both to the individual and to others.
- The extent of help available and the sustainability of that help.
- Changing circumstances over time.

Examples of treatment strategies underpinned by the above factors are provided in Table 10.5. However, it is important to acknowledge the suggestions provided in Table 10.5 are not a blueprint for occupational therapy treatment, given the individual set of circumstances which each person will present with and the requirement to respond appropriately.

Some of the extrinsic and intrinsic factors which shape the treatment process are now considered in more depth.

Development of a collaborative relationship with the older person

Salo-Chydenius (1994) stated that occupational therapy must be located in a collaborative relationship between therapist and the depressed individual, so that both parties are in a position to provide feedback. Mountain (1998) explored the perceptions of occupational therapy by older people who had received a service, as well as ascertaining views of assessment and treatment from the therapists themselves and from other members of the multi-disciplinary team. The research found that situations where the occupational therapist had the time to develop a relationship with the older person were considered to be the most productive by all stakeholders. However, it is far more difficult to develop any form of relationship with an older person when the referral is for brief occupational therapy intervention only; a situation which can predominate in situations where resources are at a premium. While it has to be accepted that this can be necessary, the benefits to the individual of more intensive work is irrefutable. The study by Mountain (1998) found that confusion and concern about the purpose and outcomes of treatment was greatly reduced if not extinguished if the older person felt that they were in partnership with the therapist over their treatment. Having full understanding of the reasons for referral and the subsequent treatment plan was also influential in determining extent of cooperation. Even if it appears that the older person may have difficulty comprehending, explanations must be given to support the recommendation of certain treatment strategies. Paradoxically, longer-term work with these older people places far greater demands upon the occupational therapist. This form of working requires a flexible approach to take into account changing needs, and a willingness to manage more intractable, difficult behaviour which may surface over time. Good practice guidelines for treatment are summarized in Table 10.6.

Maintaining an empathic approach

Occupational therapists must understand and be empathic to the person's problems, while at the same time maintaining an objective approach (Salo-

Table 10.5. Examples of treatment strategies.

Presenting problems	Further information needed	Possible treatment approaches
Physical limitations; frailty	• Which tasks are considered to be essential. • Longstanding routines. • Extent of help available and its perceived adequacy/acceptability. • Leisure and social needs. • Risk factors.	• Teach new strategies to cope with daily occupations. • Provide assistive equipment and teach usage. • Advise on safety and preventative measures to reduce risk. • Adapt longstanding interests or explore new pastimes.
Physical illness	• Attitudes towards illness and mortality. • Effects of illness upon physical functioning in short and longer term. • Extent of help available and for what. • Current and future needs for additional support.	• Lifestyle advice taking illness into account. • Teach strategies to cope with daily tasks. • Provide assistive equipment if indicated. • Adopt a flexible approach to take account of health changes day to day and over time. • Explore leisure interests which can be achieved within physical abilities. • Advise on safety and preventative measures to reduce risk.
Changes in life circumstances, e.g. bereavement, moving home, entering residential care	• Emotional and practical implications of life changes. • Any life skill deficits. • Extent of help available. • Willingness to accept available help.	• Time to express feelings and adjust to new circumstances. • Teach new life skills or revisit neglected skills if indicated. • Explore new opportunities for leisure occupations and accompany/support as necessary. • Work with other carers so they are able to participate in the rehabilitative process.
Social isolation/ solutions. alienation	• Existing care network. • Reasons for isolation and its duration. • Previous lifestyle and interests. • Any interplay between isolation and ability to undertake occupations. • The lifestyle the person would like to have and what is feasible. • Social outlets in the locality.	• Take time to explore the dynamics of the situation before offering. • Offer new opportunities for socialization if indicated but resist developing a social relationship. • Assess occupational function and suggest strategies/interventions as indicated. • Undertake a staged approach towards the introduction of new occupations, e.g. by initially supporting new social situations.

Continued.

Table 10.5. Continued.

Presenting problems	Further information needed	Possible treatment approaches
Lack of motivation	• Explore reasons for lack of motivation. • Assess risk factors resulting from lack of motivation. • Previous lifestyle and interests. • Help available and the sustainability of that help.	• Spend time talking with the person about their current circumstances and past lifestyle. • Devise small strategies to improve activity levels with the person, but be prepared for setbacks. • Mobilize other health/social care agencies, particularly if problems threaten health and safety. • Be prepared to offer longer term support. • Support informal carers to continue caring. • Solve any problems which can be addressed through practical strategies
Co-existence of other interventions, mental health problems	• Examine occupational function and explore possible reasons for any observed and reported difficulties. • Listen to the views of the user and their carers.	• Observe the impact of solutions offered. • Be alert to the emergence of other problems over time. • Refer to other agencies for advice and specialist help as indicated.
Home situation poses risks	• Assess possible hazards in the home. • Observe abilities in self care tasks. • Determine the older person's views of the risks they are taking and the options available if risk is admitted. • Consider the risk the person poses to both themselves and others through observation and discussion with carers. • Explore extent of easily accessible help from both formal and informal sources	• Suggest strategies to improve safety. • Offer extra social care provision if available and indicated. • Suggest day care options which provide an alternative to home during the day. • Offer advice and support to carers.

Table 10.6. Treatment: good practice guidelines.

- Devise the treatment programme in partnership with the older person and their carers.
- Ensure that the treatment programme takes into account the entirety of the person's needs rather than being confined to a medical speciality.
- Incorporate the needs of the carer into the treatment by offering support and advice, teaching rehabilitative skills if appropriate and recommending respite care before a situation reaches crisis.
- Work with the entire care network of the older person, being alert to changes in the context of current and future needs.
- Be alert to over-compliance and non-compliance, encouraging a continuing open dialogue about success of treatment as perceived by the service recipient.
- Be flexible and respond to changing needs within the treatment programme.
- Encourage new skills as well as the maintenance of longstanding occupations.
- Be prepared to engage with the person and their carers on a long-term basis.
- Understand the legislative framework and responsibilities within it.
- Measure the outcomes of treatment.

Chydenius 1994). This is a potentially problematic area for all those working with older people with mental health problems. While we may have been depressed and will have certainly been physically ill during our life, health and social care professionals will have only experienced older age through interacting with and observing others. It is also too easy to become less sensitive to the problems of this group of older people and to overlook some of the strengths of older people (Table 10.1). Over-involvement is equally undesirable, as this clouds ability to make objective decisions. There will be needs which cannot be met and problems which cannot be resolved. Working with older people has not been widely acknowledged as demanding specialist training on the part of occupational therapists. However, a reiterated theme in the book edited by Mackay *et al.* (1995) is the need for both pre- and post-registration interdisciplinary training on the part of all professionals working with people who present with complex needs. It is also evident that occupational therapists must develop knowledge which is located in the needs of older people, fostering an approach which is empathic while at the same time objective. Therefore to maintain a quality service located in the needs of the older person and their carer, training is recommended for occupational therapy as a specialism and within the context of multi-disciplinary team delivery.

Encouraging engagement in purposeful activity

Salo-Chydenius (1994) stated that it is important for depressed people to engage in purposeful activity and explore new ways of thinking and acting. What purposeful activity is for older people warrants careful consideration. The synthesis of research evidence by Burton (1989) demonstrated that maintaining a quality lifestyle in older age extents beyond the ability to perform necessary tasks. It includes involvement in leisure and social occupations which are meaningful to the individual. We are not the same; some of us are sociable and like to spend time with others whereas others prefer their own company. Some people will wish to retain longstanding interests while others will gain pleasure from experimenting with new pursuits, an example being the increasing use of the Internet by older people. Despite overwhelming evidence to the contrary, health and social care professionals often adopt a very limited view of the social and recreational needs of older people once they enter the service system. Through discussions with older people with mental health problems, it was evident that while some enjoyed the traditional activities provided through day care, it was an anathema to others (Mountain 1998). Once more, this underscores the requirement for careful assessment of the occupational status and needs of the individual and the devising of a treatment plan in response. There can also be benefits in the establishment of small treatment groups to meet specific needs for a limited time. The Cochrane Library of systematic reviews contains an number of studies which demonstrate the health gains to be made from group interventions, and in particular those delivering exercise and health promotion to identified individuals.

Strategies to limit risk

One of the presenting problems shown in Table 10.5 is that of a risky situation within the older person's home. Ensuring speedy but safe discharge using information provided through risk assessment is perceived to be an important role of occupational therapy. What needs to be given equal emphasis is the interventions which occupational therapists can provide to limit risk so that it is both acceptable and manageable for the older person and their carers. A Cochrane review of interventions to reduce falling in older people (Gillespie *et al.* 1997) recommended that health screening of older people deemed to be at risk should be followed by interventions to reduce environmental factors. Wynne-Hartley (1991) studied patterns of risk taking in older age through 150 individual and group interviews with independent older people. Further data was collected through 80 questionnaires. The research found that where risk was evident, older people were willing to act upon advice and modify their behaviour. There was more of a problem with situations which were not as overtly risky. The previously quoted research evidence on the volition, habituation and performance of older people described by Burton (1989) and the study of Wynne- Hartley (1991) provide important insights for the occupational therapist who has to try and manage a potentially risky situation. It particularly emphasizes a joint approach to solving the problem with the older person.

> Most older people do not wish to make radical changes either in their place or style of living. What is required, therefore, is practical guidance in identifying potential problems and hazards and advice in how these may best be overcome. This should be supplemented by functional but attractively styled aids to easier living. (Wynne-Hartley 1991, pp. 28).

Assisting caregivers

Working with older people with depression demands that the occupational therapist works with their carers. Furthermore, this can extent to working with family and friends who are providing care as well as relatives. As well as being potentially large in number, the nature of the problems experienced by older people can change over time. Both these factors can lead to big demands upon informal carers as well as upon health and social care professionals. Given that working with older people with mental health problems is often challenging for trained staff, the strain which family and friends can experience cannot be over emphasized. This is underscored by research which revealed that 40% of 287 carers of older people were ill or disabled themselves, and over half were spouse carers (Levin *et al*. 1994). In the early 1990s working with carers was promoted through groups for carers run by professionals. However, questions have been raised about the value of such groups (Joice *et al*. 1990) and there has been a move towards a more individualized approach. This has been fostered by the implementation of the Carers' Recognition and Services Act (1995) in 1996. This gives all carers right to a community care assessment of their own needs provided the person they are caring for has been assessed. The needs of the carers of older people are well documented and include being provided with information about the illness and about available services, being able to access services like home support, day and respite care and advice and advocacy (Barnes 1997, Department of Health 1997a).

Occupational therapists have a real contribution to make here which is not always adequately recognized (Mountain and Moore 1996). All carers should be involved in, and kept informed about the occupational therapy assessment process, particularly if this may result in hospital discharge. Some carers may benefit from an approach which involves them in the rehabilitation process. Once again, the needs expressed by the individual carer and the person they are caring for should shape the interventions offered to them by the occupational therapist. An example of the requirement for heightened awareness of the demands upon carers was where the partner of an older lady with depression used visits by the occupational therapist as an opportunity for respite for himself (Mountain 1998). While this might have met his needs to a certain extent, it raises the question of whether the demands of caring and desirability for respite had been raised by any of the involved health and social care professionals.

Interface with the legislative framework

It is vital that occupational therapists have a clear understanding of the legislative framework within which they and their colleagues work, taking it into account during assessment and treatment. This need is being emphasized with the move towards jointly commissioned and provided services. In these instances occupational therapists and others are being required to work across traditional health/social care boundaries, with an understanding of both health and social care legislation being a necessity.

The two main mandatory processes which involve older people with mental health problems are:

- The care programme approach (CPA), introduced in 1991. This involves the assessment of the health and social care needs of the person, the construction of care plans to meet those needs, designating a key worker for each person and regular reviews of the plan (Social Services Inspectorate and the Department of Health 1995). The lead for this process is taken by Health agencies.
- The Social Services led processes of assessment for community care and care management implemented in 1993. Carers have a right to be assessed providing that the person they care for is also assessed.

The Department of Health acknowledge the overlap between these two processes and suggest that

> The complementary principles of the health service care programme approach (CPA) and that of social services' care management should be applied to older people according to locally agreed procedures.'(Department of Health 1997a, pp. 18).

Occupational therapists can be designated key workers for a care programme, and in some social services departments, the care manager role will be taken by an occupational therapist. The occupational therapist as a care manager is being promoted in situations where they are the most involved professional (College of Occupational Therapists 1999). However, in all situations, fulfilling the requirements of these mandated processes should still be at the heart of occupational therapy assessment and treatment. Older people with a complex range of problems admitted to hospital will require community care upon discharge. Therefore, as well as predicting safety upon discharge, assessment of functional abilities while an inpatient should also feed into arrangements for community care. This demands that occupational therapists always communicate fully with community workers. Once the person returns to the community, all professionals have an on-going responsibility to monitor arrangements to ensure that any interventions offered within the care package are meeting needs. Sustaining a quality occupational therapy service is important and the important ingredients of this are summarized in Table 10.7.

Table 10.7. Sustaining a quality occupational therapy service: essential ingredients.

- Continuing professional development; ideally with other professions and agencies.
- A robust understanding of the normal ageing process and the adaptations individuals are required to make.
- Successful working relationships with other disciplines within the same organization and from other agencies.
- Ability to deliver training and provide ongoing support to others engaged in the delivery of rehabilitations.

Outcomes of occupational therapy

One of the most important, but testing questions for all health and social care workers is whether their interventions are effective. This is particularly problematic in areas of practice where traditionally there has been little investment in research and development activity and where several interventions may be provided concurrently by a potentially large number of professionals. Moreover, outcomes will be different for service users as opposed to commissioners and managers. There is a body of research which points towards the effectiveness of occupational therapy and other rehabilitative interventions with older people, and the policy focus upon rehabilitation is leading to more research activity. A meta-analysis of the effectiveness of occupational therapy for older people by Carlson *et al.* (1996) is contained within the Cochrane library of reviews of effectiveness. The aim was to assess the effectiveness of occupational therapy in the domains of physical health, ability to carry out activities of daily living and mental well being. Analysis was conducted on 14 studies of older people with a variety of physical and mental health problems. Unfortunately, the diversity of the studies included in the analysis does not enable any more than a generalized statement about the proven benefits of occupational therapy with older people. The Cochrane reviewers note that more studies are required to look at effectiveness of occupational therapy for specific groups of older people. An earlier study by Priddy et al. (1988) used the Comprehensive Occupational Therapy Evaluation (COTE) (Brayman and Kirby 1982) to measure the effectiveness of a specifically designed occupational therapy group treatment programme to 12 older people with mental health problems receiving inpatient care over a 4–month period. The study found that participation was linked with significant improvement in interpersonal behaviour (this construct including independence, cooperation, self-assertion and sociability).

While the results of these studies are encouraging, the extent of demand for evidence of effectiveness means that occupational therapists must also routinely measure the outcomes of their interventions. Several of the assessment instruments shown in Table 10.1 can be reapplied to provide a measure of change over time. There are other outcome measures which can also be used with older people with depression, and in some cases their carers. Sealey (1998) provides a list of commonly used outcome measures in occupational therapy practice in the UK and provides advice on use of outcome measures as part of the audit process.

Further treatment considerations

A reiterated theme throughout this chapter is the complexity of the problems experienced by older people with mental health problems and the challenge this presents to occupational therapists and others who work with them.

There are a number of additional factors which should also be taken into account during the assessment and treatment processes.

Multi-disciplinary treatment delivery

In common with management of risk, all the other goals of treatment described in Table 10.3 cannot be achieved by the efforts of occupational therapists in isolation. The requirement to work in partnership with colleagues within the same organization and with workers from other agencies cannot be over emphasized. If the care networks of older people are to be the starting point, occupational therapists will find themselves working collaboratively with agencies which they might not usually come into contact with, for example the church, housing and community workers and members of the primary health care team. Hernan (1994) discusses the relevance of a team approach in the undertaking of assessment and treatment, and in the nurturing of a positive attitude towards ageing. However, it cannot be presumed that this style of working is automatic; Hernan emphasizes the need for preparation for team work through a programme of teamwork education,

> Concurrent with attitudinal awareness, the team's knowledge of gerontology . . . geriatrics, and interdisciplinary teamwork skills is also a crucial factor in planning care for older persons' (Hernan 1994, pp. 203).

Obtaining accurate views of extent of available care

If occupational therapy treatment is to be provided in a timely manner which is relevant to the occupational needs of the person and their carers, it will involve appropriate agencies and individuals in the treatment plan. This necessitates taking account of the involvement of all informal carer givers, working with them and supporting them as necessary. Occupational therapists must also foster relationships with other statutory care providers so that care can be delivered across the health/social care divide and care gaps can be identified. To achieve this, an accurate view of those providing care at any one time must be obtained. An exploration of the networks of care of older people with depression and other functional illness (Mountain 1998) revealed big discrepancies between what was described by the older people, what was documented in their case records and what was recorded by occupational therapists in their clinical notes. The older people tended to describe a far greater number of formal and informal care givers, often with a completely different view of who was the most important care giver. One lady's son was described as being her main care giver when in fact he had returned to lodge in her house and was creating demands upon her! Such differences could be tracked down to two main problems; firstly, that all professionals were not spending long enough talking to the older people and clearly ascertaining who was involved and secondly there was a tendency to interpret next of kin as being the main carer.

The message is clear; if carers are to receive adequate assistance in the manner previously described, and all professionals are to avoid both duplication of effort and care gaps, it is vital to determine exactly who is involved and in what capacity at any one time. Moreover, given that the older person will usually be able to provide an expert view of their care, this network must be checked with them for accuracy at regular intervals.

Managing difficult behaviour

Older people rarely question the decisions made by professionals. A lifetime of respect for authority figures can make it difficult for them to voice fear, distress and annoyance to about service delivery to providers. As a consequence, they are most often compliant, seeming to agree with the plans devised by the professional. However, interviews with older people (Mountain 1998) demonstrated that even though the person might appear to agree with the occupational therapist, they made measured decisions about the advice and assistance they were willing to accept and what they were not. Decisions about take-up of advice and services were frequently governed by the acceptability of existing routines and available assistance.

Another form of compliance noted was for the older person to agree with a pre-arranged plan of treatment. However, when it was time to put the plan into action, the person would refuse to participate in activities which the therapist understood were agreed.

Part of Mr M's treatment included cookery sessions but during interview, he was quite clear this was not relevant to his home routine and he was going to continue to eat sandwiches at home.
'Well, I tell you why I don't cook at home and then you'll understand. I get my groceries on Wednesday, 7 o'clock. I start breaking into them on Saturday morning. The simple reason is I come here (day hospital) on Thursday during the day, on Friday I go to day centre and Saturday, Sunday, Monday I don't go anywhere so I make sandwiches ... so I don't need to cook do I?'
Mrs W allowed the occupational therapist to show her how to use the washing machine, but admitted to the interviewer that she would not use it due to the assistance she was already receiving with laundry.
'I didn't bother because well I thought I get it done every Wednesday.'

While 'inappropriate compliance' in its various forms is not overtly disruptive, it is a symptom of treatment which is not meeting needs. Furthermore, such behaviour can be destructive in that it blocks the delivery of what could be more successful treatment. To try and avoid inappropriate compliance the occupational therapist must spend time with the older person to determine what they perceive their occupational needs to be, approaching the discussion without an agenda. If existing strategies are successful, why ask the older person to make changes? It may be more appropriate to concentrate upon another aspect which may lead to improved life quality. It may be that the treatment plan was too ambitious and the person was not able to achieve the goals. If so, the occupation needs to be deconstructed into achievable steps as identified by the service user.

A further rather worrying finding which came out of the same study was that some very needy individuals were not receiving the range of services they required to support them. There were two reasons identified out of the study. The first was that the person had a partner and it was presumed that they would provide care even though they were also elderly. This is substantiated by larger scale research (Wenger 1984). The second was that the person was perceived to be difficult by care providers, with intractable problems which could not be treated. One of the challenges of working with older people with mental health problems is the commitment to try and improve their quality of life, in the case of occupational therapists through fulfilling needs for occupation. While rapid assessment and referral to other services might be an easier option in that it avoids having to manage difficult needs, the reality is that these people benefit most from longer term occupational therapy treatment.

Understanding cultural differences

Culture shapes opinions and values, determines life experiences and influences expectations. Anticipation of death is one example; when asked about quality of life in old age, Sikh elders will embrace death, quite different to the Western conceptualization. Comprehending the ways different cultures undertake self care and other occupations and expectations about retaining independence or being looked after in older age are critical when working with any older person. Research into the self care needs of Hindu elders conducted by Gibbs and Barnitt (1999) found that the concept of independence was an anathema to this cultural group. The overwhelming assumption was that they will be looked after by family members; a belief that could only be fulfilled if the family were available to do so. White (1998) undertook an ethnographic study to explore the health needs of older people from a number of diverse ethnic backgrounds, drawing the following conclusion:

> Occupational therapists who provide health promotion and disease prevention services to minority elders can be more effective if they become sensitive to cultural as well as individual differences in treatment planning and implementation. (White 1998, pp. 1).

A future role for occupational therapists

Changes in the structure of health and social care delivery, together with a growing realization of the benefits of rehabilitation is leading to shifts in the role of occupational therapists working with older people with depression.

Health promotion and prevention

Lambert (1998) described a role for occupational therapists in lifestyle adjustments which promote health. In the early 1990s Nocon raised the potential contribution of occupational therapists in assessment of those aged 75 years and over in primary care (Nocon 1992, 1993). The policy emphasis on preventative strategies together with significant shifts in patterns of delivery of rehabilitation services into primary and community care settings should enable the development of the health promotion and preventative role of occupational therapy (Seymour 1999). For older people with depression, dimensions of this new role could include:

- Aiding detection of depression through assessment of occupational engagement in primary and community care settings, for example as part of the 75 years and over assessment in primary care.
- Provision of community-based activities which promote well being, for example physical exercise and health promotion.
- Preventative rehabilitation to promote independence and allay or delay the cumulative effects of increasing physical frailty, for example through home assessment and the provision of advice and aids and adapta tions to prevent accidents.

Supervising generic workers to undertake rehabilitative interventions

Policy interest in rehabilitation is leading to unprecedented demand for the services of occupational therapists and other rehabilitation specialists. Government demands for the introduction of jointly commissioned and provided services (Department of Health 1997b) has led to a proliferation of new styles of service across the country. The demands of services which cross the health/social care divide will require all occupational therapists to make changes to established patterns of working. A review of intermediate care for frail older people to inform service development (Mountain 1997) observed that changes are required to meet projected staffing needs. It was recommended that therapists adopt a training role so that less qualified generic workers are able to undertake aspects of the rehabilitative role. This is a culture shift for a profession where the importance of direct clinical contact is still most frequently perceived to be paramount. There is no doubt that in the future this training and supervisory role will be enhanced by the use of technology, one example being that of tele-rehabilitation. This involves the use of technology, and in particular video conferencing as a means of maintaining close access to specialist services and professional help. It can therefore be used to support unqualified generic staff in the delivery of rehabilitative interventions within a person's own home and is being used successfully in other countries, and in particular in the USA.

Key points

- The role of the occupational therapist with older people with depression is a specialist area of work; to deliver an effective service, all professionals need extra training and ongoing support.
- Some of the recommendations for practice provided appear deceptively simple, but if occupational therapists are to make a real difference to these older people, the realities of trying to improve quality of life through occupation and lifestyle adjustments are extremely demanding.
- We all need to have a life which extends beyond undertaking necessary functional tasks to having enjoyment and stimulation. The challenge for occupational therapists is to enable this through assisting individuals to maintain necessary occupations and, if appropriate, encouraging them to develop new skills in older age.

References

American Association of Occupational Therapists (1995) Position Paper: Purposeful Activity. *American Journal of Occupational Therapy*, **49**, 1081–1082.

Banerjee S. (1993) Prevalence and recognition rates of psychiatric disorder in the elderly clients of a community care service. *International Journal of Geriatric Psychiatry*, **8**, 121–131.

Barnes, D. (1997) *Older People with Mental Health Problems Living Alone: Anybody's Priority?* DoH and SSI.

Brayman, S.J. and Kirby, T. (1982) The Comprehensive Occupational Therapy Evaluation (COTE) Scale. In *The Evaluative Process in Psychiatric Occupational Therapy*, edited by B.J. Hemphill. Slack Inc., New Jersey, USA. pp. 211–216.

Burton, J.E. (1989) The model of human occupation and occupational therapy practice with elderly patients. Part 1: Characteristics of ageing. *British Journal of Occupational Therapy*, **52**, 215–218.

Carlson, M., Fanchaing, S.P. , Zemke, R. and Clarke, F. (1996) A meta analysis of the effectiveness of occupational therapy for older persons. *American Journal of Occupational Therapy*, **50**, 89–98.

Clark, F., Carlson, M., Zemke, R., Frank, G., Patterson, K., Ennevor, B.L. *et al.* (1996) Life Domains and adaptive strategies of a group of low-income well older adults. *American Journal of Occupational Therapy*, **50**, 99–112.

College of Occupational Therapists and Association of Directors of Social Services (1999) *Meeting the Challenge: Occupational Therapy for the Community.* COT, London.

Department of Health (1997a) *The Health of the Nation: a Handbook on the Mental Health of Older People.* DoH, London.

Department of Health (1997b) EL(97) 62, *Better Services for Vulnerable People.* DoH, London.

Devereaux, E. and Carlson, M. (1992) The role of occupational therapy in the management of depression. *American Journal of Occupational Therapy*, **46**, 175–180.

Dickie, V. (1998) Clinical Interpretation of the unpackaging of routine in older women. *American Journal of Occupational Therapy*, **52**, 176–178.

Eakin, P. and Baird, H. (1995) The community dependency index: a standardised assessment of need and measure of outcome for community occupational therapy. *British Journal of Occupational Therapy*, **58**, 17–21.

Finlay, L. (1997) *The Practice of Psychosocial Occupational Therapy*. Stanley Thornes Press, Cheltenham.

Fisher, A.G. (1995) *Assessment of Motor and Process Skills*. Three Stars Press, Fort Colins, Colorado, USA.

Gibbs, K.E. and Barnitt, R. (1999) Occupational therapy and the self-care needs of hindu elders. *British Journal of Occupational Therapy*, **62**, 100–106.

Gillespie, L.D., Gillespie, W.J., Cumming, R., Lamb, S.E. and Rowe, B.H. (1997) Interventions to reduce the incidence of falling in the elderly. *Cochrane Library Systematic Reviews*, **3**, 1998.

Godfrey, M. and Moore, J. (1996) *Hospital Discharge from the Perspectives of Users, Carers and Hospital Staff*. Nuffield Institute for Health, University of Leeds.

Green, S. (1995) Elderly mentally ill people and quality of life: who wants activities? *British Journal of Occupational Therapy*, **58**, 377–382.

Hernan, J. A. (1994) Teamwork in programs for older persons. In *Teamwork in Human Services*, edited by Garner and Orelove, Butterworth Heinemann.

Joice, A., Thomson, M. and Glynn, A. (1990) Carer support groups: meeting the needs of carers and staff. *British Journal of Occupational Therapy*, **53**, 136–138.

Jonsson, H., Kielhofner, G. and Borell, L. (1997) Anticipating retirement: the formation of narratives concerning occupational transition. *American Journal of Occupational Therapy*, **51**, 49–56.

Kielhofner, G. (1985) *A Model of Human Occupation*. Williams and Wilkins, Baltimore, USA.

Kielhofner, G. and Nicol, M. (1989) The model of human occupation: a developing conceptual tool for clinicians. *British Journal of Occupational Therapy*, **52**, 210–214.

Kielhofner, G., Henry, A.D. and Walens, D. (1991) *A User's Guide to the Occupational Performance Interview*. The American Occupational Therapy Association Inc., Bethesda, USA.

Lambert, R. (1998) Occupation and lifestyle: implications for mental health practice. *British Journal of Occupational Therapy*, **61**, 193–197.

Law, M., Baptiste, S., Carswell, A., McColl, M.A., Polotajko, H. and Pollock, N. (1994) *Canadian Occupational Performance Measure*, 2nd edn. Canadian Association of Occupational Therapists.

Levin, E., Moriarty, J. and Gorbach, P. (1994) *Better for the Break*. NISW Research Unit.

Ludwig, F.M. (1997) How routine facilitates wellbeing in older women. *Occupational Therapy International*, **4**, 213–228.

Mann, A., Graham, N. and Ashby, D. (1984) Psychiatric illness in residential homes for the elderly: a survey in one London borough. *Age and Ageing*, **13**, 257–265.

Mackay, L., Soothill, K. and Webb, C. (1995) *Interprofessional Relations in Health Care*. Edward Arnold, London.

Mountain, G. (1997) *Services for Physically Frail Older People: Developing a Total Service Approach within an Intermediate Care Framework*. Nuffield Institute for Health, University of Leeds.

Mountain, G. (1998) An investigation into the activity of occupational therapists working with the elderly mentally ill. Unpublished PhD Thesis, University of Leeds.

Mountain, G. and Moore, J. (1996) *What do Occupational Therapists Working with Older People Do?* Nuffield Institute for Health, University of Leeds.

Nocon, A. (1992) *GP Assessments of People aged 75 and Over*. Rotherham FHSA.

Nocon, A. (1993) GP's Assessments of People aged 75 years and over: identifying the

Need for Occupational Therapy Services. *British Journal of Occupational Therapy*, **52**, 123–127.

Priddy, J.M., Sewell, H.H. Lovatt, S.B. and Jones, T.C. (1988) The effectiveness of an occupational therapy program in an in-patient geriatric setting. *Physical and Occupational Therapy in Geriatrics*, **6**, 63–73.

Salo-Chydenius, S. (1994) Application of occupational therapy in the treatment of depression. *Occupational Therapy International*, **1**, 103–121.

Sealey, C. (1998) Clinical Audit Information Pack: a resource pack to assist occupational therapists with clinical audit and clinical effectiveness. COT, London.

Seymour, S. (1999) Occupational therapy and health promotion: a focus on elderly people. *British Journal of Occupational Therapy*, **62**, 313–317.

Social Services Inspectorate and the Department of Health (1995) *Social Services Departments and the Care Programme Approach: an Inspection*. DoH, London.

Stewart, S. (1999) The use of standardised and non standardised assessments in a social services setting: implications for practice. *British Journal of Occupational Therapy*, **62**, 417–423.

Wenger, G.C. (1984) *The Supportive Network: Coping with Old Age*. NISW, London.

White, V.K. (1998) Ethnic difference in the wellness of elderly persons. *Occupational Therapy in Health Care*, **11**, 1–15.

Wilcock, A. (1998) Occupation for health. *British Journal of Occupational Therapy*, **61**, 340–350.

Wynne-Hartley, D. (1991) *Living Dangerously: Risk Taking, Safety and Older People*. Centre for Policy on Ageing, London.

Social treatments in care and depression

Alan Butler

Introduction
A model of life events
Social networks and intimate relationships
The role of the family
Bereavement
Finances
Accommodation and relocation

Introduction

As other authors have noted in this text depression is very common among older people but frequently undetected (Goldberg 1985). The prevalence is particularly high among those older people already suffering either chronic physical illness or a disabling condition. Because of this those providing some form of social care are either knowingly or unknowingly dealing with a large number of older people suffering from depression. For example it is estimated that 26% of those people receiving home care (home help) are clinically depressed (Banerjee 1993) whilst the figure rises to 40% for those in local authority care homes (Ames 1991).

Whilst this picture may be rather gloomy what those working in this field must hang onto is the fact that most older people with depression will get better (Murphy 1983) – for a more detailed review see Chapter 3. Therefore the strategy should be one of supporting and maintaining the older person whilst one of the physical or psychological treatments discussed in this book begin to have their effect. There is some evidence that by the manipulation of various social factors, an intervention may be mounted in order to mitigate the depressive symptoms. It is also possible that by maintaining or changing various social conditions and remaining alert to the needs of older people some depression may be preventable.

In this chapter I intend to explore some of these social interventions and indicate how they might be orchestrated in order to maintain an older person. In order to do this I have chosen to focus upon the following areas:

- a model of life events;
- social networks and intimate relationships;
- the role of the family;
- bereavement;
- finances; and
- accommodation and relocation.

A model of life events

In her excellent monograph *Preventive Strategies for Older People* (1999), Mary Godfrey reports that a number of studies (Green *et al.* 1992, Roberts *et al.* 1997) have demonstrated a relationship between what may be termed social isolation and the onset of clinical depression in older people. In part this reflects the wider picture in that the preventive effects of having a partner or somebody to confide in have been noted in many studies involving the general population. Livingstone and colleagues (1990), examining an inner city population of older people, demonstrated that older people who were not currently married or living on their own, were the ones more likely to suffer from depression.

The best known sociological model for the aetiology of depression is that of George Brown and Tirril Harris (1978) in their work initially conducted in Camberwell, South London. Whilst their model is most frequently used as a way of exploring and explaining depressive symptoms in women it does offer us insights into possible ways that the symptomatology may develop in older people – the majority of whom will be female. Their work was further developed in old people by Murphy (1982). The starting point for their analysis is an acceptance that stress and particularly stressful life-events play an important part in the precipitation of mental illness. Brown and Harris trace the origins of their own work back to the classic studies of Eric Lindemann (1944) when he explored the reactions experienced by people suffering a grief reaction after a bereavement. The concept of a life event as a stressor was established. This concept was developed by Dohrenwend and Dohrenwend (1974) when they concluded that life events could be typified as anything that disrupts or threatens to disrupt usual daily activities. However, they broadened the concept by positing that not only events regarded as negative, by the participant, needed to be taken into consideration. For example, moving house or acquiring a new job must be regarded as significant life events even if they were being eagerly looked forward to by the person involved in the changes. Returning to our focus upon older people, we may regard retirement in exactly the same light. Even if stopping work were keenly anticipated and well planned for it would still constitute a major life event. Paykel (1978) made another major advance when he began to categorize life events according to their meaningfulness and demonstrate that the qualitative differences between events could be shown to precede various psychiatric disorders.

Brown and Harris (1978) established that 'severe' life-events were almost four times more likely to have occurred to depressed women patients than to the normal control group. They concluded that certain other factors in the individuals background might also mitigate or exacerbate the impact of the life event. They constructed a model of the social aetiology of depression which I believe has relevance for our greater understanding of the problem amongst older people. The model has three dimensions:

Vulnerability factors

These factors were seen to leave the individual particularly vulnerable at the time of a major life-event. Of relevance to older people were things such as lack of employment outside the home and the absence of a close confiding relationship with a partner.

Provoking agents

These refer to factors that are operating in the person's contemporary life such as a bereavement or the presence of a serious or chronic illness.

Symptom formation factors

Factors which mainly impact upon the severity and form of the depression. These include previous depressive episodes and age: those above 50 being particularly vulnerable.

This model was developed in order to account for depression in women aged between 18 and 65 but it does seem to me to have a resonance for much older people of both genders. As a group they experience many major life events:

- bereavement;
- loss of function;
- illness; and
- enforced relocation, etc.

Because of their economic circumstances, old people frequently lack the resources to counter the problems they face. The importance of social support, loneliness and life events as risk factors for depression in old age has been confirmed by Murphy (1982).

The model provides a framework of understanding and is suggestive of how we might orchestrate either a holistic intervention or preventive strategy utilizing a multi-disciplinary team work approach.

Social networks and intimate relationships

One of the key factors appearing to prevent or mitigate depression in the Brown and Harris work (1978) was the availability of somebody to confide in. There seems no reason to believe that a close confidante and a rich social network should be any less important in older people. Oxman *et al.* (1992), in seeking to explore the relationship between depression and social networks in older people, examined a cohort on two occasions, with a time gap of 3 years. They demonstrated the importance of the following factors in accounting for the different levels of depression by using a multiple regression analysis:

- disability;
- role of the family;
- a close confidante available;
- extent of emotional support;
- loss of spouse; and
- presence of tangible support.

Although disability seemed to be the factor contributing most to the variance, the others do give us valuable clues as to how we might seek to maintain an older person whom is seen to be vulnerable. At the very least a poor social support, and a denuded social network, would appear to be maintenance factors for depression. Henderson and colleagues (1986), in an Australian study, have also produced evidence which suggests that elderly depressed people report a lack of richness in their social contacts.

Dorothy Jerrome (1993), employing qualitative techniques of interviewing drawn from social anthropology, has explored the importance of intimate relationships to a group of older people. She characterized such relationships in the following way:

- emotional intensity;
- self-disclosure; and
- a high degree of personal involvement

Many of her respondents paint a vivid picture of the importance of these relationships to their well being and enjoyment of life. Jerrome (1993) has illustrated just how important close relationships are in later life. They provide older people, in her view, with some of the following:

- A sense of continuity with the past.
- Help in socializing into some of the new roles that come with old age. For example, that of grandparent, or widow.
- They provide a 'natural' reminiscence group, helping the individual to keep in touch with their past and exercise their memory.
- A chance to continue to maintain or develop skills.
- Moral and practical support.
- Simple companionship.
- A forum to discuss family problems and put them into some perspective.

Such work merely serves to underline what we have learned, in recent years, about the importance of friendships and the social network that we have access to in the general maintenance of good physical and mental health. The late Mark Abrams (1980) invokes the analogy of our own lives being like a convoy moving through time. As individuals we are flanked by a number of supportive relationships – parents, wider family, friends – which provide us with support and assistance, helping us to cope with loss and change as we make progress through our lives. Berkman and Syme (1979), in their work on relationships and physical health, concluded that an involvement in a rich social network was the single most powerful predictor of survival.

The role of the family

When people reflect about social networks, in later life, the first thing they tend to think about is the role of the family. A popular view is that the family has declined as a source of support for older people. However the evidence tends to belie this point of view. Many older people live close to their children, see them regularly and receive a good deal of informal support. However, the changing circumstances of the family and other social changes, not all of them negative, have created new and challenging situations for some.

- More people now survive into 'old' old age. This means that ones children might be 75 or 80 years old themselves.
- More people now divorce and separate – but more remarry, some very late in life.
- More people are geographically mobile – but new methods of communication make keeping in touch easier. Intimacy at a distance is possible.
- More older people now live on their own. However, in part this reflects the exercise of a positive choice.

The pattern of family relationships tend to echo those to be found in younger cohorts. Continuity of activity and familial contact is much more common than the notion that becoming old or retiring marks a profound change from how things were in the past. For example, in married couples, the husband usually sees his wife as a close confidant. However, for the wives an adult child, or a same sex friend is more likely to assume the role. Most of this familial contact and networking will continue to flourish for many older people without the need for any intervention on the part of the health or welfare services. However, for some people there may be the need to support this activity or even replicate or recreate it. The statutory services may be able to provide some of the following:

- a lively, well-run day centre;
- educational and activity-based courses;
- good, easy to access, transport;
- leisure and recreational facilities geared to the older citizen; and
- streets that older people feel are safe to walk in.

The non-statutory sector, such as voluntary and religious organizations, may also play an important part in helping to support older people and provide opportunities for people to meet and socialize. Sometimes, if family life becomes particularly fraught or tangled, more formal interventions such as family therapy or counselling may prove to be necessary and helpful (Blazer 1982, Benbow *et al*. 1990).

Bereavement

One obvious life event that older people experience more frequently than most of us is bereavement and the grief that follows. Bereavement has for a long time been recognized, in all age groups, to be associated with an increased risk of death, raised levels of physical disease and depression (Parkes 1975). And yet it remains a relatively under explored area with regard to older people. As Norman and Redfern (1997) note, normally grieving elderly people may exhibit the following picture:

- depressed mood;
- loss of interest;
- poor concentration;
- poor sleep;
- poor appetite;
- weight loss; and
- agitation.

It is often a difficult judgement as to when a 'normal' grief reaction becomes something more serious such as clinical depression that will require specific treatment. Jacobs and Lieberman (1987) suggest the following three key indicators:

- pervasive loss of self-esteem;
- marked psycho-motor retardation; and
- suicidal ideas.

Others have suggested that a temporal marker be used – symptoms persisting over 6–12 months, for example (Norman and Redfern 1997). A recent monograph by Andrew Long *et al*. (1999) thoroughly reviews the relationship between bereavements, suffered in later life, their impact upon the individual and the coping strategies and interventions that might helpfully be deployed. In their extensive review of the literature they identified the following key risk factors as being of special significance when considering depression following a bereavement:

- The young elderly (65–74 years) are more susceptible to depressive symptoms, in both the short term (up to 12 months) and the longer term (3 years plus).
- Education and income seem to play a protective role in bereavement outcome.

- Depression prior to bereavement was a major risk factor for depression following the bereavement.
- The death of somebody one is closely attached to (spouse, parent, child) is more significant for depression than the death of grandchild, sibling or friend. The death of a spouse being particularly potent.
- The suicide of a spouse raises the risk of subsequent depression.
- Other life events, running concurrent with the bereavement, increase the likelihood of a depressive episode.

In trying to explore the aftermath of bereavement, for an older person, two avenues suggest themselves:

- How does the individual cope and what strategies do they use? And
- What, if any, interventions might be offered to mitigate the impact of the death and try to prevent a depressive episode resulting?

Long *et al.* (1999), when considering the coping strategies adopted by older people, identified the following:

- **Personal characteristics:** Lund *et al.* (1993), following a 2–year longitudinal study, concluded that the best indicator of adjustment were 'personal resources unique to each person'. Whilst seemingly rather vague it does point to positive self-esteem and competency in tasks of daily living as being the key indicators of a favourable outcome following a bereavement. In terms of prevention this should alert us to be aware of those bereaved older people who lack basic coping skills, such as the ability to prepare a meal unaided (males seem to be particularly implicated!). They should be targeted for rehabilitation and training or perhaps supportive care or domiciliary assistance.
- **Close relationships:** The presence of close relatives or friends seems to be a good indicator of successful coping. Once again this should be borne in mind when making an assessment. A network of support through a day centre place may also be useful.
- **Personal activity:** The ability to keep busy and active is regarded as a positive indicator of adjustment. Once again the use of social welfare facilities may be indicated.
- **Beliefs:** Long *et al.* (1999) reviewed a number of studies indicating that religious belief and practice helped the bereaved to overcome their grief. Helping people to retain these links by providing transport and involving voluntary groups seems appropriate.
- **Leisure activities:** An active interest in a sport or leisure activity, particularly if it is one shared with others, seems to be associated with lower rates of anxiety and a reduction in the feelings of loneliness experienced by many following a bereavement.

The coping strategies successfully adopted by many older people to combat the effects of bereavement suggest ways in which social interventions might be mounted. Following an assessment some of the following may be considered in discussion with the person concerned:

- social clubs;
- attendance at a day centre;
- making links with voluntary and religious groups; and
- helping with transport.

There are no simple nostrums available and a good deal is dependent upon the thoughts and wishes of the bereaved older person. There is evidence that providing a support group is helpful, at least in the short run (Tudiver *et al.* 1992), and that individual counselling, particularly if the grief appears to be complicated and unresolved, may also be of assistance. The main message seems to be that a full assessment, exploring social network, family ties, coping skills, and leisure and social activity, should always be completed when a bereaved and vulnerable older person is encountered. Any interventions can then be planned in partnership with the client.

Finances

The majority of older people do not work, they are therefore reliant upon savings or pension for their income. For most this will mean a drop in income by about half that enjoyed when in employment. Many elderly people face a future denuded of luxury and the prospect of poverty. The *Pensions: 2000 and Beyond* report noted (Retirement Income Inquiry 1996) that there is a growing disparity between those older people who are better off and those who fare badly: the very old, and single elderly women were particularly vulnerable. In 1979 The British government severed the link between the level of state pension and the index of prices or earnings (whichever was the greater). Indexation solely to prices has resulted in a steady erosion of the value of the state pension.

Many older people are entitled to extra state benefits to enhance their meagre pension – currently one of the lowest in Europe. A variety of funding streams such as income support; help with housing costs; disability allowances and help with heating costs, etc. are available to people in particular circumstances. But all the evidence suggests that many older people do not claim fully the benefits to which they are entitled. For example, Income Support (formerly supplementary benefit) which would not only provide cash but act as a gateway to other benefits such as free dental treatment and grants from the Social Fund, is claimed by only about a third of those entitled to make use of it (Retirement Income Inquiry 1996). There are a variety of reasons to explain this:

- lack of knowledge;
- intrusive and complex bureaucracy;
- fear of the stigma felt to be attached to being labelled a claimant; and
- procedures of disclosure required felt to be demeaning.

The DSS estimated that in 1993/4 pensioners had the lowest take up rates for housing benefit, income support and council tax benefit. Lack of money and fear about one's financial future may have a variety of effects upon the individual many of which contribute to a depressive mood, or exacerbate a depressive illness. They include some of the following:

- poor quality diet and even hunger;
- inability to heat the home;
- constant worry about bills;
- fears about future capital expenditure, e.g. the washing machine breaking down or the roof springing a leak;
- restrictions upon the ability to travel;
- limitations on socializing, visiting family and friends;
- unable to pursue hobbies;
- debt; and
- unable to get away for a break or take a holiday.

Trying to visualize just some of these factors in our own lives should give some indication as to the likely effect upon mood state. Whenever working with an older person it is imperative that their financial circumstances are explored. Claiming welfare benefits can be a highly technical business, and if the older person is agreeable, specialist expertise should be sought. Sources of help may include:

- the benefits agencies themselves;
- a specialist welfare rights worker within a Social Services Department;
- the Citizens Advice Bureau;
- voluntary agencies such as Age Concern.

It is easy to envisage how the lack of money acts as an accelerator to some of the other factors that I highlighted earlier in this chapter, increasing social isolation, reducing mobility and undermining the ability to cope. Many of the other interventions that we may make can be so easily negated if the older person is living in penury.

Accommodation and relocation

Where older people live is of vital importance to their well-being. In spite of a widely held stereotype, very few live in institutional settings (5%). The majority (90%) live in ordinary domestic housing similar to the rest of the population. A further 5% live in some form of sheltered housing – accommodation built for and with older people's needs in mind, usually with an on-site warden and an alarm system.

For some older people living in mainstream housing can be a great burden. They may have to struggle with poorly designed homes that are difficult to heat and costly to maintain. If they are owner–occupiers they may not have a mortgage still to pay but they are constantly aware of actual or potential major maintenance or repair bills.

For those in the rented sector, particularly if they have a private landlord, the problems may be those of poor housing conditions (damp, inadequate plumbing, outside lavatories, etc.). It has been estimated that about 700 000 of our older households occupy some of the worst housing conditions in England (Rolfe *et al.* 1993).

Struggling with inadequate housing and the burden of worry that may accompany that contributes to the feelings of depression and almost certainly makes bringing about an improvement to mental state more difficult. However, evidence suggests that many older people want to 'age in place' and remain in their own homes for as long as possible (Tinker 1994). To encourage and facilitate this a number of innovative schemes have been devised by housing organizations and social service departments to effect housing improvements and 'plug' into the home a wide range of supportive domiciliary services. An evaluative study for the DOE/DHSS conducted by Anthea Tinker (Tinker 1984), *Staying at Home: Helping Elderly People*, demonstrated that this was an option that many older people wanted to exercise. The housing improvements were part of a package containing statutory and informal support and were found to be a successful way of providing help and maintaining people in their own homes.

For those seeking a move to more compact, easy to manage accommodation, Sheltered Housing has proved to be a popular option. In Great Britain just over half a million people live in such a setting. Most of them rent from either a local authority or a housing association, but a small and growing number are buying into such schemes as normal owner–occupiers. As well as specially designed accommodation, able to enhance and maintain mobility in the frailer older person, most schemes have an alarm system and a resident warden on hand to offer some assistance (Butler 1983). Sheltered Housing has been seen as fulfilling a number of different roles:

- A social role: encouraging socialization and reducing isolation.
- A housing role: providing easy to manage accommodation to those wishing to down-size.
- A role in prevention: halting or slowing the slide into residential care.
- An oversight role: providing a rapid response to any emergencies that may befall an older person.

Whilst meeting the housing needs of many older people may bolster their self-confidence and feelings of autonomy, moving at any time in life, has its downside.

We know, from a number of studies, that moving house constitutes a major 'life event' (Dohrenwend and Dohrenwend 1974) with the subsequent rise in stress levels and generalized feelings of uncertainty and discomfort. How much greater when the person moving is elderly (and therefore likely to have lived in their former home a considerable number of years) and when the move may be enforced?

The 1991 census indicated that about 3% of those aged 70–74 moved during the previous year, but that this rose to 8% among the over 85s. A distinct pattern of movement emerges: those moving at or about retirement tending to move on housing grounds; whilst those in the older age groups do so because of the need for enhanced care or surveillance (Warnes and Ford 1995).

A number of researchers (Aldrich and Mendkoff 1963, Lieberman 1961, Markus *et al.* 1972) have demonstrated that relocation, in the elderly, may result in negative as well as positive effects. These include:

- increased mortality;
- reduction in activity levels; and
- increased incidence of depression.

A comprehensive reassessment of the field by Schulz and Brenner (1977) was more cautious but did suggest that the effects of relocation could be mitigated by two factors:

- the degree to which individuals are able to control and predict events surrounding the move; and
- the degree of control the individual retains over their life following the move.

There are undoubted gains to be made for some older people if they change accommodation in later life. But we need to be sensitive to the meanings attached to the move by the individual concerned. We also need to be aware of the potential downsides in terms of the relocation effect.

Those working with older people need to be sensitive to these issues, respect the individual's autonomy, and ensure that choice and control, wherever possible, should remain in the hands of the older person.

Key points

- Too often the plight of the older person, suffering a depressive episode, is seen as a narrowly medical matter. In this chapter I have tried to suggest that the individual, and their symptoms, need to be seen in the context of their wider life: their financial status; housing situation; family and friendship networks.
- The series of interventions and strategies that I have highlighted rely for their impact upon good multi-disciplinary teamwork. The clinician, by orchestrating a cohesive unit and making use of the skills owned by nurses, social workers, occupational therapists, counsellors and volunteers, among others, should be enabled to deliver a whole package of care.
- In this way the chance of delivering a successful treatment will be enhanced and the quality of life enjoyed by the older depressed patient improved.

References

Abrams, M. (1980) Transitions in middle and later life. In *Transitions in Middle and Later Life*, edited by M.J. Johnson, pp. 15-30. British Society of Gerontology, London.

Aldrich, C. and Mendkoff, E. (1963) Relocation of the aged and disabled, a mortality study. *Journal of the American Geriatrics Society*, **11**, 185–194.

Ames, D. (1991) Epidemiological studies of depression among the elderly in residential and nursing homes. *International Journal of Geriatric Psychiatry*, **6**, 347–354.

Banerjee, S. (1993) Prevalence and recognition rates of psychiatric disorder in the elderly clients of a community care service. *International Journal of Geriatric Psychiatry*, **8**, 125–131.

Benbow, S.B., Egan, D., Marriot, A. *et al.* (1990) Using the family life cycle with later life families. *Journal of Family Therapy*, **12**, 321–340.

Berkman, L.P. and Syme, S. (1979) Social network, host resistance and mortality. *American Journal of Epidemiology*, **100**, 186–204.

Blazer, D.G., (1982) *Depression in Later Life*. Mosby, St Louis.

Bowling, A. (1994) Social networks and social support among older people and implications for emotional well-being psychiatric morbidity. *International Review of Psychiatry*, **63**, 41–58.

Brown, G. and Harris, T. (1978) *Social Origins of Depression: A Study of Psychiatric Disorder in Women*. Tavistock, London.

Burn, W.K., Davies, K.N., McKenzie, F.R. and Brothwell, J. (1993) The prevalence of psychiatric illness in acute geriatric admissions. *International Journal of Geriatric Psychiatry*, **8**, 171–174.

Burns, A., Jacoby, R. and Levy, R. (1990) Psychiatric phenomena in Alzheimer's disease, III: disorders of mood. *British Journal of Psychiatry*, **157**, 81–86.

Butler, A., Oldman, C. and Greve, J. (1983) *Sheltered Housing for the Elderly: Policy, Practice, and the Consumer*. Allen and Unwin, London.

Dohrenwend, B.S. and Dohrenwend, B.P. (1974) *Stressful Life Events: Their Nature and Effects*. Wiley, New York.

Dura, J.R., Stukenberg, K.W. and Kiecolt-Glaser, J.K. (1990) Chronic stress and depressive disorders in older adults. *Journal of Abnormal Psychology*, **99**, 284–290.

Godfrey, M. (1999) *Preventive Strategies for Older People: Mapping the Literature on Effectiveness and Outcomes*. Anchor, Oxford.

Goldberg, D. (1985) Identifying psychiatric illness among general practice patients. *British Medical Journal*, **291**, 161–162.

Green, B.H., Copeland, J.R., Dewey, M.E. *et al.* (1992) Risk factors for depression in elderly people: a prospective study. *Acta Psychiatrica Scandinavica*, **86**, 213–217.

Henderson, A.S., Grayson, D.A., Scott, R. *et al.* (1986) Social support, dementia and depression among the elderly living in the Hobart community. *Psychological Medicine*, **16**, 379–390.

Jacobs, S. and Lieberman, P. (1987) Bereavement and depression. In *Presentations of Depression: Depressive Symptoms in Medical and other Psychiatric Disorders*, edited by O.G. Cameron, John Wiley, New York.

Jerrome, D. (1993) *Good Company: An Anthropological Study of Old People in Groups*. Edinburgh University Press, Edinburgh.

Lieberman, M.A. (1961) Relationship of mortality rates to entrance to a home for the aged. *Geriatrics*, **16**, 515–519.

Lindemann, E. (1994) The symptomatology and management of acute grief. *American Journal of Psychiatry*, **101**, 141–148.

Livingstone, G., Hawkins, A., Graham, N. *et al.* (1990) The Gospel Oak study: prevalence rates of dementia, depression and activity limitation among elderly residents in inner London. *Psychological Medicine*, **20**, 137–146.

Long, A., Godfrey, M., Randall, T., Brettle, A., Grant, M. and Chapman, M. (1999) *Effectiveness and Outcomes of Preventive Services for Older People: Risk Factors, Coping Strategies and Outcomes of Interventions in Bereavement*. Nuffield Institute for Health, Leeds.

Lund, D.A., Caserta, M.S. and Dimond, M.F. (1993) The course of spousal bereavement in later life. In *Handbook of Bereavement: Theory, Research and Intervention*, edited by M.S. Stroebe and W. Stroebe, pp. 126–146. Cambridge University Press, New York.

MacDonald, A.J.D. (1986) Do general practitioners 'miss' depression in elderly patients? *British Medical Journal*, **292**, 1365–1368.

Markus, E., Blenker, M., Bloom, M. and Downs, T. (1972) Some factors and their association with post relocation mortality among institutionalised aged persons. *Journal of Gerontology*, **17**, 376–382.

Murphy, E. (1982) Social origins of depression in old age. *British Journal of Psychiatry*, **141**, 135–142.

Murphy, E. (1983) The prognosis of depression in old age. *British Journal of Psychiatry*, **142**, 111–119.

Norman, I.J. and Redfern, S.J. (1997) *Mental Health Care for Elderly People*. Churchill Livingstone, Edinburgh.

Oxman, T.E., Berkman, L.F., Kasl, S., Freeman, D.H. and Barrett, J. *et al.* (1992) Social support and depressive symptoms in the elderly. *American Journal of Epidemiology*, **135**, 356–368.

Parkes, C.M. (1975) *Bereavement: Studies of Grief in Adult Life*. Penguin, Harmondsworth.

Paykel, E.S. (1978) Contribution of life events to causation of psychiatric illness. *Psychological Medicine*, **8**, 245–253.

Retirement Income Inquiry (1996) *Pensions: 2000 and Beyond*, Vol. 1. The Retirement Incomes Inquiry, London.

Roberts, R.E., Kaplan, G.A., Shema, S.J. and Strawbridge, W.(1997) Prevalence and correlates of depression in an aging cohort: the Almeda County study. *Journals of Gerontology. Series b. Psychological Sciences and Social Sciences*, **52**(b) 5.5. 252–258.

Rolfe, S., Mackintosh, S. and Leather, P. (1993) *Age File '93*. Anchor Housing Trust. Oxford.

Schulz, R. and Brenner, G. (1977) Relocation of the aged: a review and theoretical analysis. *Journal of Gerontology*, **32**, 323–333.

Tinker, A. (1984) *Staying at Home: Helping Elderly People*. HMSO, London.

Tinker, A. (1994) The role of housing policies in the care of elderly people. In *OECD, Caring for Frail Elderly People*, pp. 57–82. OECD, Paris.

Tudiver, F., Hilditch, J., Permaul, J. and McKendree, D., (1992) Does mutual help facilitate new widowers: report of a randomised controlled trial. *Evaluating Health Professions*, **15**, 147–162.

Warnes, A. and Ford, R. (1995) Migration and family care. In *The Future of Family Care for Older People*, edited by I. Allen and E. Perkins, pp. 65–92. HMSO London.

Concluding remarks

Depression in older people is common and associated with high morbidity and distress in patients and their families. It is important that patients receive a thorough medical, psychological and social assessment if this important condition is to be successfully treated. Untreated depression, particularly when associated with physical illness, is associated with an increased mortality emphasizing the importance of early and accurate diagnosis and treatment. Depression in older people responds well to treatment. However, an integrated approach that concentrates on the patient's physical health combined with pharmacological treatments, psychological approaches and social interventions is usually needed. This can only be achieved by a range of health care professionals working together and this has been the key message emphasized in this book.

Index

Page references in *italics* refer to figures; those in **bold** refer to tables